PRAISE FOR *UNOFFENDABLE*

"With his characteristic recipe of subversive humor and radical grace, Brant effectively calls all-too-easily-offended followers of Jesus to a far less grumpy witness and a whole lot less toxic faith. A good antidote to the dis-graced faith we have become all too accustomed to."

— Alan Hirsch
Award-winning author of
*ReJesus, The Shaping of Things
to Come*, and *Untamed*

"In *Unoffendable*, Brant Hansen has produced a small stick of dynamite to throw into every crowd of complaining and contentious Christians who have lost sight of what Scripture teaches about the glory of over-looking an offense. A much needed book for the times."

— Frank Viola
Author of *God's Favorite Place
on Earth* and *From Eternity
to Here*

"I'm truly excited about *Unoffendable*—not just for the greater church that often seems stuck on the Technicolor sins, but for my own heart. Brant's wisdom and stories are beckoning for me to choose wonder, gratitude, and hope over the entitlement and judgment that is so tempting to sit in."

— Charlie Lowell
Jars of Clay and cofounder of
Blood:Water

"If you choose to read this book, you are choosing to enter the danger zone. If you choose to embrace the core message of this book, you will be freed to love in dangerous ways. And if you are serious about becoming more like Jesus, truly, then devour this book ASAP and then shout 'FREEDOM!' from the top of your lungs."

— Dale Brantner
President/CEO,
CURE International

UN
OFF-
END-
ABLE

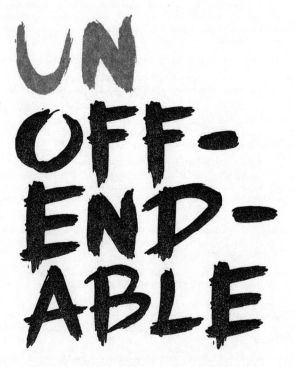

UN OFF- END- ABLE

HOW JUST ONE CHANGE CAN MAKE ALL OF LIFE BETTER

BRANT HANSEN

W Publishing Group

AN IMPRINT OF THOMAS NELSON

Published in Nashville, Tennessee, by W Publishing Group, an imprint of Thomas Nelson.

Thomas Nelson titles may be purchased in bulk for educational, business, fund-raising, or sales promotional use. For information, please e-mail SpecialMarkets@ThomasNelson.com.

Any Internet addresses, phone numbers, or company or product information printed in this book are offered as a resource and are not intended in any way to be or imply an endorsement by Thomas Nelson, nor does Thomas Nelson vouch for the existence, content, or services of these sites, phone numbers, companies, or products beyond the life of this book.

Library of Congress Cataloging-in-Publication Data

Hansen, Brant.
  Unoffendable : how just one change can make all of life better / Brant Hansen.
    pages cm
  Includes bibliographical references.
  ISBN 978-0-529-12385-5 (trade paper)
  1. Anger—Religious aspects—Christianity. 2. Choice (Psychology)—Religious aspects—Christianity. 3. Forgiveness—Religious aspects—Christianity. I. Title.
  BV4627.A5H36 2015
  234'.5—dc23   2014035483

Printed in the United States of America

*To all those who want grace for themselves
but struggle to extend it to others.*

Wait: that's everybody.

Anger is the most fundamental problem in human life.

—Dallas Willard[1]

CONTENTS

CONTENTS

1

BEING UNOFFENDABLE: THE RIDICULOUS IDEA

Okay. So this may sound like the dumbest thing you've ever read, but here goes:

You can choose to be "unoffendable."

I actually heard a guy say this at a business meeting. That is striking to me for a few reasons: (1) I'd never, ever thought about that before; (2) I *remember* something from a business meeting; and (3) I was actually invited to a business meeting.

I remember the guy saying it's a choice we can make, to just choose not to be offended.

Sure. Right, man. Choose to be unoffendable. Just—you know—choose, as if it's really just up to us.

I found this offensive.

• • •

By the way, I just looked up the definition of *offended*, and all the dictionaries say something about anger and resentment. When I'm writing about the word here, then, that's what I mean.

There's another definition, about having your *senses* affronted, or offended, but that's not the definition we're dealing with here. We just made some homemade barbecue sauce the other day, and we unanimously and immediately agreed, right then and there, that it was highly offensive. That happens.

It's the *taking* of offense, and the very presumption that I'm somehow *entitled* to be angry with someone, that I'm talking about. Surely there's got to be a place for "righteous anger" against someone, right? Surely there are times we are justified in our anger . . .

Wasn't I *supposed* to be angry at people for certain things? Isn't being offended *part of* being a Christian?

But what that guy said at the business meeting did get me thinking, because he was so obviously wrong. And besides, since I call myself a Christian person, wasn't I *supposed* to be angry at people for certain things? Isn't being offended *part of* being a Christian?

So I did what any rational, fair-minded, spiritually mature person would do: I scoured the Bible for verses I could pull out to destroy his argument, logically pummel him into submission, and—you know—win.

Problem: I now think he's right. Not only *can* we choose to be unoffendable; we *should* choose that.

We should forfeit our right to be offended. That means forfeiting our right to hold on to anger. When we do this, we'll be making a sacrifice that's very pleasing to God. It strikes at our very pride. It forces us not only to think about humility, but to actually be humble.

I used to think it was incumbent upon a Christian to take offense. I now think we should be the most refreshingly unoffendable people on a planet that seems to spin on an axis of offense.

Forfeiting our right to anger makes us deny ourselves, and makes us others-centered. When we start living this way, it changes everything.

Actually, it's not even "forfeiting" a right, because the right doesn't exist. We're told to forgive, and that means anger has to go, whether we've decided our own anger is "righteous" or not.

● ● ●

I sense a lot of people think this idea is stupid, and they don't agree with me on this. And I sense this because lots of people say, "That idea is stupid, and I don't agree with you on this."

I've got antennae for subtlety like that. I pick up on things.

Plus, lots of the Christian literature out there says I'm wrong.

Typical: This entry from an online devotional, dealing with anger. The writer gives what I think is the reigning understanding: anger's often just what we need!

> There is also a positive, even essential, side to anger. I doubt that we ever accomplish anything fruitful when anger isn't part of our motivation, on a certain level at least.[1]

We don't ever accomplish *anything* fruitful without anger? Including, say, writing devotionals?

Here's another example of how we retrofit actual scripture with our current embrace of anger-culture:

Ephesians 4:26 NCV
When you are angry, do not sin, and be sure to stop being angry before the end of the day.

Ephesians 4:26 MSG
Go ahead and be angry. You do well to be angry—but don't use your anger as fuel for revenge . . .

Did you catch that? I love Eugene Peterson—the guy who wrote *The Message*—but sheesh! "You do well to be angry"? That's not in the original, folks. That's an updated version. Hope you like it better.

It's remarkable that Peterson does this, considering that just a couple of sentences later, Paul wrote, "Do not be bitter or angry or mad" (v. 31 NCV). And somehow, from this, we get "You do well to be angry"?

Honest question: Why do we decide to read the Bible that way when it comes to this issue?

And another question: Why, when I talk about anger on my radio show, do so many believers instantly go to the scripture about "In your anger, do not sin," and then skip the rest of the paragraph? Why ignore the context? *Do not be bitter or angry.*

Paul was saying, clearly, that, yes, we will get angry; that happens; we're human. But then we have to get rid of it. So deal with it. Now. We have no right to it.

Another fair question, and one you're likely asking: But isn't God allowed to hold on to His anger? Doesn't Jesus get angry?

My well-read, thoughtful, theologically nuanced response to this is, "Well, yeah, of course."

God is "allowed" anger, yes. And other things, too, that we're not, like, say—for starters—vengeance. That's

Yes, we will get angry; that happens; we're human. But then we have to get rid of it.

His, and it makes sense, too, that we're not allowed vengeance. Here's one reason why: We stand as guilty as whoever is the target of our anger. But God? He doesn't.

For that matter, God is allowed to judge too. You're not. We can trust Him with judgment, because He is very different from us. He is perfect. We can trust Him with anger. His character allows this. Ours doesn't.

God loves you and thinks you're special, but no . . . you're not God.

● ● ●

We won't often admit this, but we *like* being angry. We don't like what caused the anger, to be sure; we just like thinking we've "got" something on someone. So-and-so did something wrong, sometimes horribly wrong, and anger offers us a sense of moral superiority.

That's why we call it "righteous anger," after all. It's moral and good, we want to think.

Problem is, "righteous anger" directed at someone is pretty tricky. It turns out that I tend to find Brant Hansen's anger more righteous than others' anger. This is because I'm so darn right.

I'm me. I tend to side with me. My arguments are amazingly convincing to me.

But inconveniently, there's this proverb that says, "You may believe you are doing right, but the LORD will judge your reasons" (Prov. 16:2 NCV).

So it's not just me. We all, apparently, find ourselves pretty darn convincing. *Of course* my anger is righteous. It's righteous because, clearly, I'm right, and they're wrong. My ways seem pure to me. Always.

> **The thing that you think makes your anger "righteous" is the very thing you are called to forgive.**

In the moment, everyone's anger *always* seems righteous. Anger is a feeling, after all, and it sweeps over us and tells us we're being denied something we should have. It provides its own justification. But an emotion is just an emotion. It's not critical thinking. Anger doesn't pause. We have to stop, and we have to question it.

We humans are experts at casting ourselves as victims and rewriting narratives that put us in the center of injustices. (More on this in a bit.) And we can repaint our anger or hatred of someone—say, anyone who threatens us—into a righteous-looking work of art. And yet, remarkably, in Jesus' teaching, there is no allowance for "Okay, well, if someone really *is* a jerk, then yeah—you need to be offended." We're flat-out told to *forgive*, even—especially!—the very stuff that's understandably maddening and legitimately offensive.

That's the whole point: *The thing that you think makes your anger "righteous" is the very thing you are called to forgive.* Grace isn't for the deserving. Forgiving means surrendering your claim to resentment and letting go of anger.

Anger is extraordinarily easy. It's our default setting.

Love is very difficult. Love is a miracle.

Today I read an article in *Inc.* magazine about anger and Martin Luther King Jr. The author quoted King's autobiography, where he wrote, "You must not harbor anger." But that's not all. Even when attacked, wrote King, we should love our enemies.[2]

The author did the usual thing, and spun King's statement into something of an endorsement of anger, saying we should just make sure we use anger constructively. Fair enough, but I disagree with the author. A couple of things are remarkable about this article, one being that the author purports to *agree* with Martin Luther King Jr., while saying something nearly the opposite! At a minimum, it's much less radical, and far less poetic.

King says, "I must not harbor anger," and the author says, "I agree; let's use our anger constructively!"

I think we do this with Jesus all the time. We take something like "Love your enemies," and "Pray for those who persecute you," and tack on, "But, really, holding on to anger is justified."

We do it with the apostle James, who, in the Bible, said point-blank that anger does *not* produce the kind of righteousness God wants in us: "The anger of man does not produce the righteousness of God" (James 1:20 ESV).

We do it with Paul, when we read one of his many lists of sins, like Colossians 3:8: "But now also put these things out of your life: anger, bad temper, doing or saying things to hurt others, and using evil words when you talk" (NCV).

We don't like the "anger" part. We think that when he said to put anger "out of your life," he really meant "except when it's constructive." I've yet to hear us apply that logic to the rest of his teaching in that verse: "Get rid of your evil words—except when it makes sense," or "Rid yourself of evil words—except when they really had it coming."

Let's admit it: we like anger—our own anger, that is—at some level. We're just so . . . justified.

● ● ●

Upon hearing my ideas on anger, a radio listener told me, "I don't get it. Shouldn't we be angry at those guys in the news who beat up homeless people?"

Here's what I think, given that we're to "get rid of all anger": Anger will happen; we're human. But we can't keep it. Like the Reverend King, we can recognize injustice, grieve it, and act against it—but without rage, without malice, and without anger. We have enough motivation, I hope, to defend the defenseless and protect the vulnerable, without needing anger.

Seek justice; love mercy. You don't have to be angry to do that. People say we have to get angry to fight injustice, but I've noticed that the best police officers don't do their jobs in anger. The best soldiers don't function out of anger.

Anger does not enhance judgment.

Yes, God is quite capable of being both just and angry, but if I'm on trial in front of a human judge, I'm sure hoping his reasoning is anger-free.

Some people think I'm nuts when I talk about this, when I say we're not entitled to our anger. And maybe I am. At first, I hated this idea too. The thing is, now I'm hoping I'm right, because life has become so much better this way, and I think I can understand Jesus more.

2

EVERYONE'S AN IDIOT BUT ME

This book isn't an autobiography, but it's worth telling you where I'm coming from. By my very nature, I'm a Pharisee. I'm a rules guy. I'm also naturally very resentful.

What's more, I was raised in conservative churches, the son of a preacher man. I am very practiced at seeming righteous and impressing people with my outward piety. I know how to play the religion game. You should also know, given the nature of this book, that I'm not a pacifist, and neither my conservative nor my liberal friends would say I'm particularly liberal, theologically or politically. Further, I'm not advocating that there is no wrong or right, or that sin doesn't exist.

Choosing not to take offense is not about simply ignoring wrongs. If someone, say, cuts in front of you in line, you can address the situation. You don't have to simply accept it. But you can act without contempt, anger, and bitterness.

Yes, there is right and wrong, and what Jesus has done for us is the antidote to both fuzzy-minded relativism and self-righteous religiosity. According to the radical teaching of Jesus, I stand as guilty, morally, as any other sinner, period.

Whatever anyone's done to me, or to anyone else, I stand just as guilty. People have lied to me, but I've lied too. People have been unfaithful to me, but I've been unfaithful too. People have hurt me, and I've hurt them. I get angry toward murderers, and then here comes Jesus, telling me if I've ever *hated* someone—and I have—I am the murderer's moral equal.

No one likes to hear this. We want to think people are worse than us. It's one of our favorite pastimes.

Don't believe me? An experiment: Go to a mall food court, grab a chicken kabob or something, sit down, and listen to the conversations around you. Compare how often people are telling stories about hurtful, wrong things other people did, versus confessing hurtful, wrong things they, themselves, have done.

We're brilliant at this. Geniuses, really. Would that the Nobel Committee had a prize for this.

Happens in traffic all the time. The other day, I was leaving our gym's parking lot, waiting in my car to turn left, sitting toward the middle of the exit, and some guy pulled in quickly and almost hit me. My mental response: *Geez, that guy's an idiot.*

And then, this very morning, I was the one entering the lot, and some guy was sitting there waiting, in the exact same place I'd been, and I thought, *Geez, that guy's an idiot.*

Geez. That guy's an idiot. I've done the *exact* same thing he was doing . . . but *that* guy's an idiot. And the other guy who did *exactly* what I was now doing? Yeah, that guy's an idiot too. "That" guy is always wrong, because he's always that guy. I'm always *this* guy.

In other words: Everybody's an idiot but me. I'm awesome. Go me.

(Inspiring quote for you to highlight and tweet, immediately: "Everybody's an idiot but me. I'm awesome."—@branthansen)

Moral of the story: The other guy is always the jerk. Many times in my life, I've vocalized, in traffic, something like, "Man, what a jerk." I can't remember ever, not once, saying, "Man, *I'm* a jerk." Why? Because I'm a victim. My intentions are pure. Other people are the perps. I'm never a perp.

It's as natural as breathing, but that doesn't make it right. It's as universal as eating, but that doesn't make it right either. Because whatever they did? *We're just as guilty.*

I'm not entitled to my anger against them, and I'm not entitled to *think* I'm entitled to my anger. And yet, many tell me that we can, even should, keep our anger for a time. I ask, "How long are you allowed?" and I've heard the same answer, many times: "You can keep it for a little while."

Sounds reasonable. Sure. Absolutely. But merely "reasonable" isn't what we're going for here. We want to follow the gospel, wherever it takes us. God has a way for us to live—a humility that He has called us to—and it's the way we humans happen to really flourish.

It's how *you* will flourish.

* * *

I hear this objection too: "What about being angry at *sin*, Brant? Of course, we're supposed to be angry at sin."

It's probably worth noting that, usually, when this question is asked of me, it's about something more specific. By "sin," we mean, *other people's* sin.

Are we to cling to anger at their sin? God took out His wrath on Jesus for other people's sin. And I believe Jesus suffered enough to pay for it, and my sin too. I'm so thankful for that. He will deal with others' sin; it's not my deal.

That's a huge relief. Again, life is better this way.

As for my own sin, well, He says He's taken that sin away from me as far as the east is from the west (Ps. 103:12). I suppose I could whip up some anger, but I'm honestly just stuck feeling grateful right now.

What's more, for those who still want to make anger a nutritious part of their spiritual breakfasts: in the Bible's "wisdom literature," anger is always—not sometimes, *always*—associated with foolishness, not wisdom. The writer recognized that, yes, anger may visit us, but when it finds a residence, it's "in the lap of fools" (Eccl. 7:9).

Let that sink in. When anger lives, that's where it lives: in the lap of a fool.

Thinking we're *entitled* to keep anger in our laps—whether toward the sin of a political figure, a news network, your dumb neighbor, your lying spouse, your deceased father, whomever—is perfectly natural, and perfectly foolish.

Make no mistake. Foolishness destroys.

Being offended is a tiring business. Letting things go gives you energy.

And while I thought the idea of choosing to be "unoffendable" was ludicrous, I've tried it. And I'm not perfect at it, but I'm much, much better than I used to be. I just let stuff go. I go into situations thinking, *I'm not going to be offended. No matter what.*

I can let stuff go, because it's not all about me. Simply reminding myself to refuse to take offense is a big part of the battle.

Truth is—and you already know this—most of the time, whatever it was that we were taking personally, *it really didn't have to do with us.* Some people are rude, or selfish, or whatever, and we were just in the wrong place at the wrong time. It happens. We can take it personally if we want . . . but *why*?

Author Frank Viola believes that Christians are more easily offended than anyone else.[1] I think Frank is brilliant, but I actually don't think that's true. In my experience, people—all people—thrive on being offended. It makes us feel more righteous to get aggravated at the behavior of other people. And that's true of all of us, not just religious folk.

> I can let stuff go, because it's not all about me. Simply reminding myself to refuse to take offense is a big part of the battle.

Shoot, we get offended by the behavior of people we don't even know. We'll go out of our way to do it, consuming news to hear what outrageous thing some celebrity did or said. Our whole culture does this. Taking offense is a national sport. And as for Viola's claim that Christians are the worst, well, I live near San Francisco, and while it's largely a post-Christian culture, there are plenty of things one can do or think that the culture there will find terribly offensive.

It's actually a very long list. It's just a different list.

Natural as this is, Jesus came along and gave us a distinctly supernatural, and radically better, way to live. (Oddly, working in Christian media, I hear from a lot of people who are all about living a "radical" Christian life. *Radical* is a great word. But when it comes to something as radical as, say, dropping our right to offense or anger . . . ? No thanks.)

It's true that sometimes people try to offend us, and they're intentionally hurtful and spiteful. And yet, there Jesus is, on the cross, saying, "Father, forgive them. They don't know what they're doing."

A fair question, then: Is that same Jesus living in and through me, still saying that?

●　●　●

And here's another tough question: Are we really, honestly aware of just how little we actually know about other people?

When it comes to human motives, deciding *why* people do the things they do—you know, who's righteous and who isn't— we're actually worse than clueless, because while we're being clueless, we're simultaneously under the impression that we're brilliant.

In what must surely be one of the most ignored passages of the Bible, Paul wrote this two millennia ago:

> As for myself, I do not care if I am judged by you or by any human court. I do not even judge myself. I know of no wrong I have done, but this does not make me right before the Lord. The Lord is the One who judges me. So do not judge before the right time; wait until the Lord comes. He will bring to light things that are now hidden in darkness, and will make known the secret purposes of people's hearts. Then God will praise each one of them. (1 Cor. 4:3–5 NCV)

That's amazing. Think about what Paul was writing there: He doesn't know anyone's motives. *Not even his own.*

Even if his own conscience was clear, that didn't make him innocent. Paul was aware of his own inability to judge himself. He couldn't be trusted. So, he said, leave the judging up to God. He'll sort it out in the end.

This can't be glossed over. Think about how taking this to heart could deflate our own anger, even before it takes hold. *We have no idea what is in someone else's heart.* We don't know the backstory. We don't know what's happening in his mind. We don't know how her brain works. We think we do, sure, but we don't.

So let's review:

God knows others' private motives. We don't.
God knows our private motives. We don't.
We think we can judge others' motives. We're wrong.

We should abandon our "right" to anger, simply because we can deceive ourselves so easily. And—this is stunning—get this: if you fancy yourself a reasonable, fair-minded person, you may be in *particular* peril of fooling yourself.

Dan Kahan, a Yale law professor, recently led a study that found that our passions and biases undermine even basic reasoning. The study showed that people who are normally very adept at math are suddenly unable to solve a problem when the obvious answer conflicts with their political beliefs.

And it's not as if the "smartest" people were able to do better at solving the problems. In fact, the researchers found that the better the people were at math, the *more* apt they were to try to avoid the actual answer.[2] (This applied to both liberals and conservatives, by the way.) Instead of changing our beliefs to match reality, we often just rearrange reality, in our heads, to match what we want.

Yet another wrinkle: when there are two "sides" to a story, we tend to think the first one we hear is the right one. I learned this, of course, by watching *The People's Court* after school every day. I always thought the plaintiff had a great case . . . until I heard the other side.

This bias is universal. It's not new, either. Check out Proverbs 18:17: "The first one to plead his cause seems right, until his neighbor comes and examines him" (NKJV).

Life is full of conflicts, disputes, differing perspectives . . . and in all of those, guess whose perspective I hear first? That's easy: mine. I establish a story line, and I can get angry before I even hear the other side, which is yet another reason to be very suspicious of ourselves.

So let's have the guts—and the humility—to believe what the Bible says about us, and what the research shows us. We simply can't trust ourselves in our judgments of others. We don't know what they're really thinking, or their background, or what really motivated whatever they did.

And since we don't know, let's choose ahead of time: we're just not going to get offended by people.

If I don't need to be right, I don't have to reshape reality to fit "The Story of My Rightness." That makes life much easier, and makes us much more peaceful, and even fun to be around.

Oh yes, the heart is deceptive. And that calls for humility above all else, because my heart isn't deceptive because it fools other people.

It's deceptive because it fools *me*.

3

SIX BILLION RINGS

There's something powerful, and incredibly compelling, about someone who refuses to be offended.

My friend Michael is a very evangelical Christian. He decided to open a coffee shop in the downtown of a city with a large university, in the middle of a thriving arts scene. He opened it right in the middle of the usual assortment of feminist bookstores and hipster apartments. He planned to bring in big-name Christian musicians for concerts and feature evangelical speakers.

The local paper wrote about him and his wife and their purchase of one of the most significant buildings in the downtown area, as well as their evangelical plans for the coffeehouse.

I winced when I saw the article. I had other friends in that neighborhood and knew none of them would welcome this development. In fact, before Michael bought the building, it had hosted the community's biggest arts event of the year. It was an exhibition to benefit AIDS research, and it featured local art—some of the very intentionally "transgressive" variety.

We could see the culture war coming.

One of the exhibit organizers saw Michael on the street and asked how things were going with the remodeling of the building. He also mentioned to Michael that, of course, he and his team would be looking for a new place for their exhibition this year.

Michael said no, they wouldn't need to do that. They could still have the event in his building. They were welcome.

The guy was stunned. "Really," he said, "that's not necessary." He knew Michael wouldn't want this kind of crowd in his coffeehouse.

Michael told him that not only were they welcome, but he'd pay for all the catering. He'd buy the wine and hors d'oeuvres.

They couldn't believe it. What about the art that Michael would surely find offensive?

Michael said they were welcome anyway. And they were.

My wife and I went to the exhibit and, sure enough, we didn't like some of the art, for a variety of reasons, though much of it was stunningly thoughtful and beautiful. But Michael had told the event organizers that he didn't need to appreciate all the art. He just wanted to make them feel at home.

Instead of being evicted, by Christians, from the best location for the exhibit, the artists were welcomed. Michael and his wife met everyone at the door. He dressed in a tuxedo and offered everyone chocolate-covered strawberries. Live music filled the room. It turned out to be the best exhibit the group had ever had.

That was Michael's style. He hugged everybody. He talked freely about Jesus, but people didn't mind. He told me he would just talk to people about the goodness of God, because he knew, deep down, that everyone is yearning for a God like that.

An acquaintance of ours who ran a business nearby was open about her distaste for Christians and her affinity for Wicca. But she loved Michael, and would listen to him talk about Jesus. She said she knew he was different because when she'd drop by his coffee shop, in her all-black apparel, he'd run over and hug her.

She knew he wasn't offended by her. He loved her, and not just as a project. He *liked* her, even.

Christians in the community wanted Michael to be offended, to draw another line in the sand. You're supposed to get angry, and maybe even picket those kinds of people. Michael fed them strawberries. He was less interested in what some Christians thought than he was about his chance to introduce "offensive" people to a God who loves us all and wants to change us all.

Love, as it turns out, covers a multitude of offenses. It sure opens doors.

And hearts too.

● ● ●

Your life will become less stressful when you give up your right to anger and offense.

And by the way, if you don't, you're doomed. So there's that too.

C.S. Lewis wrote:

One man may be so placed that his anger sheds the blood of thousands, and another so placed that however angry he gets he will only be laughed at. But the little mark on the soul may be much the same in both. Each has done something to himself which, unless he repents, will make it harder for him to keep out of the rage next time he is tempted, and will make the rage worse when he does fall into it. Each of them, if he seriously turns to God, can have that twist in the central man straightened out again: each is, in the long run, doomed if he will not. The bigness or smallness of the thing, seen from the outside, is not what really matters.[1]

Forgive in the big things and the small things. Don't take offense.

In fact, the stuff that usually might offend us is a huge opportunity! Jesus told us we will be forgiven as we forgive others.

> So what if—just dreaming out loud, here—Christians were known as the people you couldn't offend?

Fact is, most of us don't get *that* many opportunities to forgive. Once I realized that, traffic went from being an exercise in anger to "forgiveness practice." Life is so much better that way.

I used to be scandalized by others' moral behavior. I'm just not anymore. It frees up a lot of mental space, and we probably need more of that, to pause and reflect on what matters in life. Sure, I've used my free mental space for baseball statistics and Duran Duran lyrics, but I can do better. So can you.

It's not that I think that potentially offensive behavior is "right" or "good." Not even close. It's just that it's not about *me*. I'm not going to be threatened or scandalized by someone else's immoral behavior.

So what if—just dreaming out loud, here—Christians were known as the people you couldn't offend?

Yes, we get angry. Can't avoid it. But I now know that anger can't live here. I can't keep it. I can't try it on, can't see how it looks. I have to take it to the Cracks of Doom, like, *now*, and drop that thing, much as I want to wear it awhile. (Note: I'm really going to try not to use four thousand *Lord of the Rings* analogies in this book. I may fail.)

I'm not entitled to anger, because I'm me. I can't handle anger. I don't have the strength of character to do it. Only God does. We can trust Him with it. Jesus gets angry, but His character is beyond question, so He is entitled.

We all think that we deserve to carry anger, but it will destroy us unless we let it go. We have to deny ourselves, die to ourselves, and surrender ourselves.

Whatever it takes.

Anger is like the One Ring. But the *Lord of the Rings* analogy breaks down here: There's not a single, hyperdestructive One Ring to be thrown into the cracks of Mordor.

There's, like, six billion.

Drop yours.

4

ARTISTS SEE THINGS

O ffense obscures our vision. Removing offense enables us to see people in wonderful, new ways.

I once worked part-time as a baseball announcer for minor-league teams and, occasionally, during March, for major-league spring-training games. I was the guy they'd call to fill in for a friend of mine named John, who's an absolutely brilliant announcer, and a very well-known radio pro too.

John is a class act. He arrives at each game impeccably dressed, highly organized, and briefcase in hand. That's how he rolls. He's polished. He's polite. He's clean. He's smooth. He's successful. He's also a professing Christian.

Seated next to John at each game is his polar opposite in the behavior department. Bill (I changed the name here) is a grizzled former player whose life has taken some twists and turns for the worst. He's boisterous and foul. His language is remarkably crude. Pornographic, even.

He's very tough to take.

As I worked with Bill, filling in for John, I wondered, *Wow! How does John, who's even more take-charge, blunt, and straight-laced than I am, deal with this guy? And it's night in, night out. I can't imagine how he handles this.*

When profane Bill found out I was friends with buttoned-down John, he gave me my answer. I braced myself. I'll leave the profanity out, but it went something like this:

"You're friends with John, really?"

"Oh, yeah."

"You know what? I got something to say about that guy. That guy, John, is . . ." He paused. Then, momentarily, he continued: "A couple of weeks ago, you know what he did? He brought in a plaque he had made for me. It was the magazine cover from back in the day, me and my teammates. He had an original cover put in the plaque, and he gave it to me to honor me."

Bill was actually tearing up.

"You know what?" he went on. "That guy is really good to me. And he just treats everyone the same up here. All of us the same. The interns, me, the stadium manager, every-body. He just treats us all like he loves us."

Several seconds passed before he finally concluded, "I still can't believe he did that for me."

I e-mailed John after the game and told him that I'd just heard one of the greatest compliments ever, and it was about him: *he treats us all the same.*

John simply refused to be offended. He was free to love Bill just the way he was.

My instinct, and I'm sure the instincts of many in Bill's life, was to tell Bill to shut up, or at least watch his mouth, or get his act together. Or maybe I could ignore him.

But John? John went and made him a plaque.

● ● ●

Some people are artists. They just see things better. When they look at something, they see potential outcomes. They see what could be. Like my friend Chris.

Chris was elated at his find one time, and he enthusiastically showed it to me. It was a pile of flattened cardboard boxes he'd gotten from a Dumpster. Seriously, he was overjoyed.

"This is the good stuff, my friend!" he told me. "Look at this!"

The good stuff?

I guess it was. Weeks later, he showed me a crèche he'd made, life-size: Mary, Joseph, and Jesus. It was painted with small flags from around the world, to demonstrate the relevance of Christ to the modern world in the midst of nations and wars.

When he told me it was made out of cardboard, I couldn't believe it. It looked as though it were chiseled from white stone. He'd made it from the "good stuff"—you know, from the Dumpster.

Chris is an artist. He just sees things.

John, my baseball-announcing friend, sees things too. He looks at Bill and sees Bill as he could be, as he was made to be. He's not being naive; he's being like God, "who gives life to the dead, and calls those things which do not exist as though they did" (Rom. 4:17 NKJV).

I love that. He "calls those things which do not exist as though they did."

• • •

Al Andrews is a counselor who tells a story about a real estate adventure he and his wife embarked on early in their marriage. They saw a relatively inexpensive house for sale in the newspaper, called the Realtor, and visited.

It was a disaster scene.

The "yard" was full of motorcycle parts and hadn't been mowed in, apparently, years. The agent told them, "Oh, isn't this great? With a little work, you can have a path here, and a flower bed there, and it'll be lovely."

And then they went inside. Again, disaster. A horribly ugly fireplace in the "living room" was doubling as a garage for motorcycles.

"This could be a wonderful living room!" the agent gushed. "You could pull up the carpets, get this cleaned, do this other thing, and then that . . ." And so it went, during the whole tour. It was one disaster after another, accompanied by one Realtor spin-control idea after another.

Thing is, Al actually bought the house. And a couple of years later, they had their agent friend back to their house for dinner. Sure enough, there were the path and the flower bed, and the living room had beautiful floors and a gorgeous fireplace, and the whole thing was just as she'd said it could be. Beautiful.

Al told me that he asked her, "How did you do that? How did you know? The grass was four feet tall! There was garbage everywhere! The windows were covered—or broken!"

He says her answer was simple: "Al . . . I can *see*."

• • •

God sees things we don't. He must, because He hasn't vaporized us yet. He must look at a seriously messed-up world and still see what can be done with it. He sees what it can and will be.

He apparently sees us the same way. He's not just an artist, of course, like Chris. He's also a Father. Good dads are like that. You may be a dropout, underachiever, whatever, and a good dad will still love you, but he'll push you to change, because he sees a different you ahead. He sees a finished product, an adult who uses his or her talents and is a blessing to others.

> **God sees things we don't. He must, because He hasn't vaporized us yet.**

He sees something wonderful.

• • •

And *we* can see where choosing "unoffendability" frees us to love people in risky but profound ways.

Jesus is this way with the most morally embarrassing people. You can't find a single story in the Bible where He's so disgusted, so scandalized by someone's moral behavior, that He writes him off. It just doesn't happen.

In fact, a friend recently pointed out something to me that I had never noticed or thought about before. I think it's remarkable.

In John 13, Jesus is having a last meal with His closest friends and followers. He tells them that He will soon have to leave them, and where He's going, they won't be able to follow Him.

Peter objects to this, and tells Him that he wants to follow, and that he'd even give his life for Jesus.

Then Jesus says, "Will you lay down your life for My sake? Most assuredly, I say to you, the rooster shall not crow till you have denied Me three times" (John 13:38 NKJV).

That's the end of the scene, and it's pretty chilling. The chapter ends right there.

But here's what I'd never thought about: The scene *isn't* actually over. Yes, there's a chapter break, but "chapters" aren't in the original. Bible translators added those centuries later to help us find things in the Bible.

The next chapter, John 14, starts with this:

"Let not your heart be troubled; you believe in God, believe also in Me. In My Father's house are many mansions; if it were not so, I would have told you. I go to prepare a place for you. And if I go and prepare a place for you, I will come again and receive you to Myself; that where I am, there you may be also." (vv. 1–3 NKJV)

So think about this: When Peter insists that he is even willing to die for Jesus, Jesus tells him, "No, you'll betray Me. You'll deny Me—three times. *But don't let your heart be troubled. Believe in me. I'm going to prepare a special place for you—and I'm coming back to get you!*"

Jesus wouldn't even let hypocrisy, betrayal, backstabbing, lying, and abandonment stop Him from loving Peter. He saw something in Peter that Peter could not have possibly seen himself. And sure enough, in the book of Acts, there's Peter, boldly putting his life on the line to tell people the good news about what God has done for them.

Yes, God sees things we don't. We can risk loving people—incredibly difficult, insulting people—because He loves us.

That person you find so offensive? Somehow, God sees something there. Something you don't. Ask Him what it is.

Maybe He'll show you. I bet He wants to.

5

BERT AND ERNIE
AND SATAN

Every time I read the Gospels, I keep waiting for something to happen, something specific—that keeps *not* happening. I am waiting for a certain reaction from Jesus.

When the disciples ask Him who's going to get to be His top-ranking, right-hand man in the kingdom of God, I keep thinking Jesus is going to lean in close, place His hands on His beloved friends' shoulders, lovingly look them straight in the eyes, and say, "ARE YOU *KIDDING* ME? WHAT IS THE MATTER WITH YOU? I CANNOT BELIEVE THIS!"

Doesn't happen. Jesus isn't shocked by self-centeredness. Neither is He scandalized by others' moral behavior. Ever. He knows how we are. He knows how the human heart works.

John 2 tells us, "Jesus didn't trust them, because he knew human nature. No one needed to tell him what mankind is

31

really like" (vv. 24–25 NLT). Maybe those who seek to follow Him could take that same approach.

Perhaps a big part of being less offendable is seeing the human heart for what it is: Untrustworthy. Unfaithful. Prone to selfishness. Got it. Now we don't have to be shocked.

Jesus is not a cynic. He's never scornful, hopeless, or jaded. It's purely about growing up enough to recognize just how messed up our world really is, and how messed up humans are.

On one level, I do understand why people can react with horror at war crimes, for instance. We all intuit, deep down, that something is simply not right about innocent lives being lost. And yet, anyone who reads history knows that war or murder—or injustice in general—is simply not the exception; it's the rule. Moreover, the last hundred years have given us no reason to think things are getting better.

We humans are so persistently naive about this, which is why an article in the satirical online news publication the *Onion* was so spot-on. The headline read, "Neighbors Remember Serial Killer as Serial Killer." When asked about him, his neighbors said he had always seemed like "the serial killer type of fellow."[1]

I probably don't need to unpack that, but here you go, just in case: The usual story is, "I just can't believe he would ever do something like that. He didn't seem like the type." What *is* "the type" to do something unthinkably horrible? The human heart is capable of staggering evil, and evil people rarely dress in horns and a pitchfork, even if it would make it easier for us to identify them.

This is one reason the TV show *Breaking Bad* was so brilliant. Rarely does entertainment—or literature, for that matter—so realistically show how someone, even a boring chemistry teacher, can justify his way to unspeakable crime. But that's the world as it is, according to the smartest man who ever lived, Jesus.

He knows the human heart. And so should we, so we can quit being shocked and adjust our expectations accordingly.

Perhaps you've noticed: Jesus encountered one moral mess after another, and He was never taken aback by anyone's morality. Ever. I can't find any stories (maybe you can find one?) where Jesus sees an immoral person and says anything like, "Wow! Okay. Well, that really *is* disgusting. That's just too much."

Jesus encountered one moral mess after another, and He was never taken aback by anyone's morality. Ever.

My wife, Carolyn, and I had a discussion regarding someone we both have known for many years. She said something like, "I can't believe she did that!" and I agreed. We were just amazed by this person's refusal to be honest, and—whoa! Wait a second. We "can't believe" she did that?

She has done exactly "that" for thirty years.

Now that I've noticed it, I hear this so often from our radio callers. "I can't believe my mom did this," or "I can't believe my sister would . . ."

And I ask, "Really? You can't believe it?"

I'm not the smartest guy in the world, but I propose that we shouldn't be shocked and amazed if someone who does that thing . . . you know . . . does that thing again.

So how about taking this idea to all of our experience: You really *can't believe* politicians would lie? You *can't believe* a preacher would cheat on his wife? You *can't believe* someone would try to steal from you? You *can't believe* a neighbor would set off fireworks at 2:00 a.m.? You *can't believe* a world leader would tyrannize his own people?

Are we going to live in perpetual shock at the nature of man?

●   ●   ●

My job has taught me a lot about this. Imagine speaking each week to more than six million people. That is hard enough, but throw this in the mix: it's a Christian music station, which means everything I say will be viewed through the lens of, "Did he say that the right way?"

I'm constantly offending people. And they've all got phones.

One day, we talked about the local forecast. "It'll be warmer than it should be for this time of year," I said. "Normally, the high is seventy-two, but today, a high of eighty-two."

The phone rang.

CALLER: You know, I was really disappointed to hear your forecast. It's not going to be "warmer than it should be," because God ordains the weather, and it's going to be exactly what He wants it to be today. Very disappointing.

ME: I'm sorry you were disappointed by this.

A bit later, I played my accordion on the air. Some say this is artistically offensive, sure, but it's all in fun. It's a goofy karaoke bit where people get to pick a hit from our station, or an '80s song, and then awkwardly try to sing along with me. One day, we did both.

The phone rang.

CALLER: You know, I noticed you sounded a lot more practiced when you played the '80s song.

ME: Uh . . . "Danger Zone," by Kenny Loggins?

CALLER: Yes, it was very disappointing that you didn't play the godly song as well as you play the worldly songs. You apparently don't want to practice unless it's a worldly song.

ME: Wait—so . . . I played "Danger Zone" too well?

CALLER: I'm really disappointed at what the station is doing, glorifying worldly things. You shouldn't glorify the world like that.

ME: With my accordion?

Another phone call.

CALLER: I'd just like to say, I listen from 7:00 to 8:00 a.m. every morning. And it's disappointing.

ME: I'm sorry—what's disappointing?

CALLER: I have yet to hear you say anything about Tim Tebow or his father's fantastic ministry.

ME: Actually, now that I think about it, I just happened to talk about Tim Tebow on yesterday's show, and I said something about how I appreciate his attitude when it comes to—

CALLER: Yeah, but it wasn't between 7:00 and 8:00.

● ● ●

Ask anyone who works in Christian radio, and you'll get similar stories. Being told you're "disappointing" is a way of life. It's enough to make someone quit, unless—and here's a big, beautiful *unless*—we just decide to quit being offended.

Here's an e-mail I got recently:

I have listened to your show many times, and all I can truthfully say is i know the devil smiles every time u pick up that mike! where should I start? I have heard u quote stalin, a dictator, mass murderer, and known satanist in a positive way. u actually told your listeners tattoos are not an issue . . . u are a theological mess! and i could possibly get past the "stoner bert and ernie shtick" and the coy flirtations with the women that call if u ever had one intelligent or spiritual thing to say, but u don't, u come up with mindless meaningless worldly spiritually bankrupt topics to discuss, and the other lukewarm undecided followers out there eat it up . . . what a shame. u have such an opportunity to help change lives, and you use it just like an apostate.

Yeah. And then it got worse.

This stuff happens. In truth, the flirting allegation stung a little bit. I'd never heard anyone say that before, and I don't ever want to come off that way. In person, I wouldn't know how to flirt if I wanted to. (My wife and I have always laughed about this.)

The Stalin thing was baseless, and I'm still not sure I understand the Bert-and-Ernie thing. Scholars may spend years unpacking the Bert-and-Ernie thing.

Anyway, I hope the lady who wrote that is okay. Used to be, I'd be mad about it and write something back to win an argument. (Or, another idea I toyed with, a one-sentence response: "So, should I put you down as a station supporter at forty dollars a month?")

Now, since encountering the reality of God's grace for me,

I honestly feel for her. Maybe I've just seen it all now. I'm not shocked.

It's not just working in Christian radio, either, that makes me feel like people are just broken by nature. I've worked in mainstream formats, like talk radio. I've had thousands of conversations with people, heard by millions of others. And once again, it turns out, people are judgmental and self-righteous by default. I am too.

So there's nothing exceptional about the aforementioned e-mail, except for that listener's deft combination of references to Joseph Stalin, Bert, Ernie, and Satan.

I'm not shocked anymore. I want to be like Jesus: "No one needed to tell him what mankind is really like" (John 2:25 NLT).

So humans are judgmental? Okay. Established. There are self-righteous people who self-describe as Christians, and there are self-righteous people who self-describe as atheists. They're self-righteous about different things, sure, but it's a very human thing to the core.

That caustic e-mail? I had to let it go. People are messed up. I know this because I talk to millions of them, and *I'm* messed up. This should not be daily news: *"I can't believe how crazy these people are . . ."* I've had to adjust my expectations and stop being offended.

Look, you have free will, and you *can* be perpetually shocked and offended. But be honest: Isn't it kind of exhausting?

This is not cynicism; this is living with realistic expectations— the very same understanding of our nature that Jesus has.

6

BEAUTIFUL EXCEPTIONS

And now we can get to the good part, the reason the Christian worldview is *not* cynicism: *we get to marvel at the goodness that humans often produce.*

Okay, we recognize that we humans are prone to dig in and make excuses for ourselves . . . but then you have that talk with a friend who did something to you, and he actually humbles himself and apologizes?

That's a beautiful thing.

Someone happily sacrifices her own hard-earned money to help a family in poverty?

Gaze at it.

Someone sees that you're burdened in an airport security line, and lets you go ahead of her?

Wonderful.

Someone who has every reason to be upset at you just lets the matter drop?

Pause and take it in. It's not the rule. It's the beautiful exception.

True story: A friend of mine who did not believe in God haphazardly drove her car into a road construction worker and cost him his legs. From a hospital bed . . . *he forgave her.* She now believes in God.

Stunning.

Another true story: A few days ago, there was a funeral for a friend of mine. Jerry was a doctor who served the poor in Afghanistan and in Chicago. After arriving for work at CURE International's hospital in Kabul, he was shot and killed by a rogue Afghan police officer.

I cried when I heard about Jerry's death. It still hurts. I loved him. But I cried again, in awe, when I saw his wife, Jan, forgiving his killer just a day after it happened. "We don't know the backstory," she said. And Jerry was there because he knew Jesus loves the people of Afghanistan.

Amazing.

> Yes, the world is broken. But don't be offended by it. Instead, *thank God* that He's intervened in it, and He's going to restore it.

Yes, the world is broken. But don't be offended by it. Instead, *thank God* that He's intervened in it, and He's going to restore it to everything it was meant to be. His kingdom is breaking through, bit by bit. Recognize it, and wonder at it.

War is not exceptional; peace is. Worry is not exceptional; trust is. Decay is not exceptional; restoration is. Anger is not exceptional; gratitude is. Selfishness is not exceptional; sacrifice is. Defensiveness is not exceptional; love is.

And judgmentalism is not exceptional . . .

But grace is.

Recognize our current state, and then replace the shock and anger with gratitude. Someone cuts you off on your commute? Just expect it. No big deal. Let it drop, and then be thankful for the person, that exceptional person, who lets you merge. See the human heart for what it is, adjust expectations, and be grateful, not angry.

When you see, in the midst of all this mess, beautiful glimpses of God's kingdom, defined by love, breathe it in. It's like the line from the motion picture *The Village*, where a young, blind woman risks a dangerous journey for a friend: "She is more capable than most in this village. And she is led by love. The world moves for love. It kneels before it in awe."[1]

The world kneels before love . . . in awe!

Recognize our brokenness, and then gaze at the beauty of God's manifested love and grace breaking into the world. It happened two thousand years ago, when wise men traveled thousands of miles, and you know what they did: *they knelt before it in awe.*

That's because grace is amazing. For now, grace is the exception, and it's a beautiful one.

● ● ●

Something happened a few weeks ago that I haven't been able to tell anyone except my wife. It was the most remarkable thing that's ever happened in my radio career.

There's a man who's in one of the worst, most brutal prisons in the world. It's in a nation where freedom of religion is notoriously disallowed, and this man, this prisoner, is a believer in

Jesus. He was arrested for precisely that, and he has been beaten and tortured as a result.

On a Saturday, his wife sent me an e-mail and told me that, amazingly, her husband was listening to my radio station at that very moment, from within the crowded confines of his tiny cell. Someone had smuggled in a phone, and she was holding her phone up to a radio speaker from her home in the States. "A whole group is listening, new believers, some Muslims. They're listening to whatever you say." He used to listen to our station every day and sing our songs with his kids. He was desperate to hear some music, or an encouraging word, she said. He'd been away from them for more than a year. He was worried he'd been forgotten by all but a few.

I drove to the station—about a two-minute drive—and went on the air. I couldn't say that he was listening, due to the security risk. But I mentioned him, the fact that millions of people were praying for him, and how much I respected him as a man and a brother in Christ.

I got to talk about how God sees prisoners, knows of their plight, and promises to rescue them. While the Koran never speaks of a God who loves, the God of the Bible loves prisoners so much that He identifies with them. He died between two thieves. And in Psalms, He "sets . . . prisoners [to] singing" (68:6).

"So maybe," I told my listeners, "if you happen to be listening in a prison somewhere, maybe you could sing along with this simple song . . ." I then played a remix of a song called "How Great Is Our God," in multiple languages. After that I talked more about how we have not forgotten about those in prison, then played a song called, "How He Loves," followed by another song, the one that the prisoner had last sung with his kids, when he put them to bed before leaving home.

All the while, the prisoner's wife continued e-mailing me: "He's listening! They're all listening! He's singing! I'm bawling . . . I can't stop crying. This music means so much to him."

They were disconnected after a half hour.

If you were to pick a spot on a world map and put a push-pin in the single most unlikely place on the planet where people would be singing along with "How Great Is Our God" and hearing about the love of God, it would have been at that prison and that dark, dank cell in the middle of the Middle Eastern night, where desperate men are starved for hope.

Grace has no borders. Love breaks through, and—just as Jesus said of the church—the gates of hell will not prevail against it.

But grace has no borders. Love breaks through, and—just as Jesus said of the church—the gates of hell will not prevail against it. Yes, the world is broken, and selfishness is our default setting. But that's all the more reason we get goose bumps when there's a ray of light, and we can suddenly see the kingdom from here, where things are set right.

Yes, we all deal with crazy people. Judgmental people. People who believe, deep down, that their job, after being invited into the party that is the kingdom of God, is to keep others out of the party, and then pat themselves on the back for "taking a stand." I hear from them often.

But then there are people like this imprisoned man, who, after being taken from his family, unjustly tried, and beaten senseless . . . *hugs his jailors.*

And then, standing in an empty studio, I get to play a simple song about the goodness of God. I sing along, knowing he's huddled in darkness with other outcasts, and they're singing too.

I want to seize *those* moments: the true, the pure, the lovely. Yeah, there are the "Bert and Ernie" letters, but then there's this. I opt to seize this.

When we recognize our unsurprising fallenness *and* keep our eyes joyfully open for the glorious exceptions, we're much less offendable. Why? *Because that's the thing about gratitude and anger: they can't coexist.* It's one or the other.

One drains the very life from you. The other fills your life with wonder.

Choose wisely.

7

THE WORLD'S WORST
BEDTIME STORY

Sheldon Vanauken tells a story in *A Severe Mercy* that sticks.[1] I read it once and never forgot it. In fact, I told it to my kids when they were little as a bedtime story. It's a great story, but you may think something's seriously wrong with any dad who would use this as a bedtime story. It goes like this:

There were two dogs who lived in the country. They had pretty much the ideal country-dog setting: beautiful rolling hills, lots of sunshine and romping, and a good master who was kind to them and loved them. It was the kind of life you'd love to have if you were a dog.

Gypsy was an older dog, and the young dog was named Snowball. Every day, about the same time, their master called them in for dinner. They knew to obey; that means they had to respond as soon as they heard their master's call.

One day, at the exact moment the master called them—"Gypsy! Snowball! Dinnertime!"—a rabbit ran across Gypsy's path. Suddenly, she felt a strange sensation: She wanted to ignore her master and chase after that rabbit. She was tempted. But she yielded to what she knew was right and went to dinner immediately, as she was trained.

But the next day, it happened again. And this time, she gave in to temptation. She heard her master's voice, but she decided she just wanted to chase the rabbit right now. And when she finally came for dinner, she came with her tail between her legs. She knew she had done wrong. She didn't want to do it again.

But she did it again. And again, until it became easier for her.

Soon, Snowball was able to run free, while Gypsy was now leashed. Her master was heartbroken. He loved her, but he knew he couldn't trust her anymore.

One day, the master loaded his dogs into the car to take them for a walk in the woods. Gypsy and Snowball loved the smells of the woods. When they arrived, Gypsy, now used to disobeying, took off before the master could put his leash on her. She was free! She ran and ran and ran into the woods! Free!

Her master called her name, desperately—"Gypsy! Gypsy! Gypsy!"—in hopes that she would return to him. He and Snowball searched for hours. But to Gypsy, his voice became more distant, until she couldn't hear him anymore. She was excited, but she noticed it was getting cold. The sun was going down.

Meanwhile, Gypsy's owner and master, who loved her so, cried as he put Snowball back into his car and drove home.

He never saw Gypsy again.

● ● ●

"Daaaaaaad! That can't be the end of the story! Daaaad!"

As I told you, you might think I'm pretty messed up for telling my kids that story. You may actually want to call the authorities at this time. I respect that conviction. I'll be here when you get back.

Of course, there *is* a little more to it, but not much.

I told them that the master drove home, and while Snowball missed Gypsy, Snowball resumed a wonderful life, romping through the meadows and always responding to her owner.

Gypsy lived in the woods the rest of her life. Her fur grew matted, and she was lost and alone. She missed her master's voice and the way he took care of her. She eventually had some puppies, and she told them about the master and how good he was. But they only knew some stories. They didn't know him.

The puppies grew up, and they told their own puppies about the master, but by then, no one really knew him at all.

And that's the end of the story. Vanauken tells it better, but that's how I told my kids. I wanted them to know that while I love God, and I want to be close to Him, He has given us all a choice whether or not to serve Him.

When they grow up, they'll have the option to reject God's love, to go their own way, to buy in to the idea that "freedom" exists elsewhere. Or they can trust that God's way brings us freedom. He has our best interests at heart. When God shows us how to live, He's doing so because He wants us to flourish, like Snowball.

When He says to get rid of anger, to serve others, and to die to ourselves, it's in our best interests to obey. He knows how we can thrive.

● ● ●

Maybe you can relate to this, maybe you can't, but I used to get into arguments online about stuff. I found there are two ways to handle this sort of thing.

Option 1:

4:10 p.m.	See insulting comment from Bob371 on blog.
4:15 p.m.	Stew about it.
4:20 p.m.	Craft amazingly thorough, literate, snarky reply to set Bob371 straight.
4:30 p.m.	Hit "submit" and walk away from computer, "drop the mic"–style, all smug and cool.
4:40 p.m.	Return to computer to delete my smug reply.
4:41 p.m.	See that someone has already replied to my smug reply.
4:42 p.m.	Delete my reply anyway, but write another one.
5:30 p.m.	Eat dinner with family, but distractedly, because I'm bugged by comments on blog.
5:45 p.m.	Decide it doesn't matter what people say. I was right.
5:50 p.m.	See another blood-boiling response from the Big Jerk formerly known as Bob371.
5:52 p.m.	Decide to write something sort of nice, but still, you know, making my point.
5:55 p.m.	See new comment. Someone else, whom I respect, thinks I was being a jerk in my original

comment. Respond to that person via e-mail, to apologize, but not really, because the jerk formerly known as Bob371 is a bigger jerk.

6:10 p.m. Write another comment, commence stewing about the whole thing until 1:30 a.m.

That's one way to handle it.

Option 2:

4:10 p.m. See insulting comment from Bob371 on blog.

4:15 p.m. Thank him for it; point out what I appreciate about it. If I want to continue the conversation, fine, but otherwise, it doesn't matter.

4:20 p.m. Go play *Madden NFL* with my daughter, get beat 75-0, then eat dinner with the fam and laugh about stuff.

I've learned option 2 is pretty awesome. And it's way more restful. I actually sleep better when I've chosen to be unoffendable.

Thing is, many people will agree with me, until they see what Bob371 wrote. Maybe he said something that's totally untrue, or anti-God, or immoral, or whatever—now what? My experience is that option 2 still works. I'm *still* opting for sleep. I don't control the world, I don't control Bob371, and I'm not going to cancel out every strand of thought on the Internet with which I disagree.

God is in control; I'm not. Is Bob371 a mortal threat to the kingdom? No, Bob371 is not a mortal threat to the kingdom. God is patient with Bob371.

In fact, God is patient with everybody right now. As someone who's ensconced in pop Christian culture, I'm with Annie Dillard, who marvels that God hasn't blown our "dancing bear act" to smithereens.[2] And then I come to a place like where I am sitting now, at this moment—a sidewalk café on the Cal-Berkeley campus—and can wonder over the same thing.

Is Bob371 a mortal threat to the kingdom? No, Bob371 is not a mortal threat to the kingdom. God is patient with Bob371.

Wow, is He patient with us.

Wow, I should be patient with Bob371.

Choosing to be unoffendable not only helps me sleep at night rather than worrying about my latest online "Stand for Truth"; it helps me remember that Jesus didn't even ask me to take a stand for truth on everything. He told His followers to go and make disciples. Make other followers.

And that takes patience with people. It takes me taking a deep breath and trusting that God has plans for, and even loves, the evil Bob371.

● ● ●

Here comes another story. Gird yourself. This one is PG-13 for implied church-organist violence.

I once took the high schoolers from our church to Kings Island, a big amusement park by Cincinnati. It has a giant, inexplicable facsimile of the Eiffel Tower. I told everyone to meet at the giant, inexplicable facsimile of the Eiffel Tower at 8:00 p.m. I was very insistent about this.

"Kids, you need to meet by this giant, inexplicable facsimile of the Eiffel Tower at 8:00 p.m.," I said. "Don't be late." They seemed to understand.

But one of the chaperones did not like this plan. He was the church organ player, a very round, late-middle-aged, egg-headed guy with glasses and a pocket protector, who was known for being proud of his Bible knowledge.

I could tell he did not like my plan because he grabbed my arm when no one was looking and told me, to my face, that I was being too "rough" on the kids, and that if I did it again, "I'm going to beat the **** out of you."

I found this scene odd. I was twenty-four, and kind of nerdy myself, sure, but the flabby church-organist guy was grabbing and threatening me? Right here, on this hallowed ground between the Turkey Leg Depot and Hanna-Barbera Land?

Round Organ Man thinks he can beat me up? Really? And it's because I actually have a rule about when to meet? I can't believe this! It's an insult to my leadership, and my masculinity.

Plus, he *cussed*?

I had two options for dealing with this:

Option 1: Just call my wife and laugh about it.
Option 2: Let it bother me deeply for, oh, about eight years.

I opted, of course, for option 2. That's because—and I hope I'm not being too technical here—I was stupid.

I'm serious. It bugged me for years. There are people who said I should've flattened him on the spot, but that would've been unwise. Plus, I'm not sure I could have. It would have been messy, and if people in a theme park–type environment saw two nerds flailing at each other next to the Turkey Leg Depot concession stand, they probably would've just thought, *I guess Kings Island does this every night at 7:30.*

Anyway, it bothered me for a long time, and my point is this: deciding "I'm not going to let people offend me" will make for a far more restful life.

Jesus said that if we come to Him, He'll give us rest (Matt. 11:28). I'm discovering how multifaceted that is. As a kid, when I heard He'd said that, I had no idea what He was talking about. Looking around at all the church people, it seemed to me that Jesus had sure given them a lot of stuff to do.

But as a young man, after I'd had some theological training and some time to really reflect on this . . . I still didn't understand it. Honestly, I thought maybe it meant after we're dead. *Then* we'll finally get some rest. Jesus will give us a break after a life of doing stuff. He'll help us rest in peace, or something like that.

Now I understand that Jesus was talking to a weary, religion-soaked people. They'd been given so much to do and so many rules to follow. So many rabbis had expounded so much the right ways to do things, and Jesus was saying, "My way is easy to understand. Kids understand it. It's you adults and 'experts' who like to make things complex. My teachings are simple at heart."

I love that so much. He's offering sweet relief from religious burdens. But He's doing even more than that. When we pay attention to what He's actually saying, like in the Sermon on the Mount, and actually put His principles into practice, we find life to be more restful.

Still, it's up to us. My kids are older now, but I want them to know that. They're free. God knows what's best for us. He offers peace. He offers rest. But He lets us choose.

I'm glad they remember the story, that one about the two dogs.

The part I want them to remember most: the Master is very, very good.

8

AIN'T YOU TIRED?

In this culture, if you live a restful life, you'll freak people out.

Maybe you already know this. My wife and I have tried it, and while we're very far from where we'd like to be with this, we've grown a lot. And yes, it sticks out.

I'd planned to go to law school a few years back. I took the test and got some great offers from top law schools. I didn't even want to be a lawyer, per se; I just love law, and logic, and the idea of having a career that sounds impressive.

Ultimately, after talking with some lawyer friends, I realized I'd have to completely set aside my family time once I graduated from law school. My wife talked a lot about it. We didn't want that lifestyle. I took the ego hit, went the other direction, and took a job in South Florida as a morning-show assistant.

It didn't pay much, but I had time with my family. Lots, actually. Some days, we pretty much did nothing.

And "nothing" turns out to be very countercultural.

We figured this out after we took up residence in a condo development that forms a ring around a pond. Thing was, everyone could pretty much see everyone else, all the time. Everyone's sliding-glass back doors face everyone else's.

We started getting comments from neighbors. One evening, standing by the pond, a tipsy Finnish guy (he and his wife were drinking while moving out, tired of the inhospitable hood) told me—I swear I'm not making this up—"I've looked outside and seen your family. I've watched you. And when I see your family, I don't even know why, but I think about God."

I'd never talked to him before.

"I watch you outside, and your wife, and your boy, and when you walk with your girl, and I see how your wife makes people feel—very welcome," he said. "It makes me think about God. I know that's strange."

Once, a single man, a guy named Steve, stopped by with his dog as Carolyn and I sat on our little back patio. Carolyn had talked with him some. Me, not so much. I have a long history of being shy . . . and selfish. I'm getting better.

"You guys ought to be in a museum!"

Uh . . . what?

"Seriously. You got the mom, the dad, the kids, all hanging out. When it gets dark, I can see you inside, eating dinner around the table and playing games and stuff. You ought to be in a museum somewhere! I love it!"

In our society's terms, what we did is a lot of nothing. For one, we didn't send our kids to school. Carolyn's a brilliant teacher, and homeschooling fit nicely into the rhythm of our home. I've heard the objections. One is this: "What about being 'salt and light'? What about sending your kids into the dark places to redeem them? What about the schools?"

Okay, fair enough. What about them? And while we're at it, what about our *neighborhoods*? What about not just getting mail there, but actually *living* where you live? Kids leave schools and change classes. People change churches and never see one another again. But where you live? Now, there's a bit more *there*, there.

Turns out, when you have time to do what, culturally speaking, is "nothing" (like walking the baby around, chatting with neighbors, letting the kids play together), neighbors get to know one another. It doesn't happen when everyone's at breakneck speed and then, when home, exhausted.

Nothing is quite something—a very attractive something. People long for it; even admire it. (One lawyer friend in Florida told me over coffee, "I hear what you're saying about not working like crazy to buy stuff, and I want to live like that. But—forgive me—you're the only one I know who actually lives like that.")

In this culture, "nothing" sticks out like crazy, like, say, a city . . . on a hill . . . or something. It wasn't just those two guys. Our whole neighborhood knew we were odd. *The dad's home a lot; he's walking around with his daughter, catching lizards? The mom is home a lot, too, talking outdoors with us about the ducks? They waste time together. They waste time with us. Something's odd here . . .*

So, "nothing" made a man think about God. In the United States right now, maybe that's not hard to explain. We did nothing, and nothing is shockingly out of place. Nothing means not everything, not running around infernally, not getting our kids this lesson and that, not trying to sustain a lifestyle we "want"— but not deep down.

No, Jesus' offer of rest isn't the "after-you're-dead" variety. It's a lifestyle, now, that invites other people out of the maelstrom.

So here's to nothing! And I don't want to sound cocky about it, but I can do nothing pretty well.

● ● ●

Trouble is, the current of our culture (and church culture can be even worse) is so strong in the other direction. We have to actively *choose* a way to live, because otherwise, we'll simply get swept along: hurried, stressed, status-driven, easily angered, and opting for madcap busyness without even knowing why. Living the usual way, we're prone to offense simply because people can't help but stand in the way of what we're straining to get.

Jesus tells us to resist. He tells us to deny ourselves, and He promises that will bring us the rest we're looking for. We have to be reminded of this. I hope, if nothing else, this book is a reminder in your life of just how good God is.

Here I am, writing this book, and I still need to be reminded. I have to continually think about this stuff, or I'll be caught up in anger toward someone. And then there's the simmering, the talking to others about that person, the energy it takes to justify my anger, and ultimately, the alienation from my offender. It might even be someone in my church community, or someone at work.

You know what else requires a lot of energy and isn't very restful? Quitting jobs. Ending relationships. Moving.

Anger leads to dissolution, one way or the other. Sadly, there are many side effects to my anger, and one of them includes my wife carefully putting our dishes, once again, in moving boxes.

Taking offense is so often a lot of work. It can wear you out;

but for some, it really becomes a lifestyle. We run into this in our small church community: People come to our group, and they're tremendously excited about it! They love it! They love us! It's great! And they want to share! So they tell us about their past church, and how messed up it was because of whatever, and then the church before that, and this other group they had to leave because people were doing such and such. (You've probably stopped paying attention to this sentence, but that's okay; I did too.)

Living the usual way, we're prone to offense simply because people can't help but stand in the way of what we're straining to get.

Gee. Think they'll soon find fault with us too? Of course. It's a way of life. We get offended; we get disillusioned; we leave. Over and over and over.

It's tiring to have to work through difficulties with people. But for what it's worth, I've learned it's way easier than starting over.

● ● ●

One of my friends, David, said something this morning during our church gathering that I keep thinking about. He said, "You know what? I think God is really just looking for spiritual people. That's what He's always been looking for. He will handle the rest. He wants a people who long to know Him, rest in Him, and love Him."

That can sound like a "Well, yeah, obviously" moment. But it didn't strike me that way. I've been thinking about it all day, how we love to do everything but "be spiritual." (By the way, it's not a generic "spiritual" we're talking about here. Spirituality must be "with" something or someone, just as much as romance or loyalty. What my friend is referring to is a spirituality based on relating to God through Jesus.)

American church culture, generally speaking, does not encourage this sort of restfulness. Quite the opposite, actually. Instead of inviting people out of the exhausting storm of busy lives, we add to their loads. We give them even more to do, or prompt them to feel guilty about what they're not doing.

How do I know this? I've done it. I was good at it.

●　●　●

Mike was a smart high school kid in my youth group years ago, and very conscientious, too, which explains the question he asked me one day. I think I'd just finished giving a lesson on tithing or something. He earnestly asked, "So, I get so confused with all this stuff. Can you just make a list for us so we know we're doing all the right things?"

"Great idea," I said. And that week, I made a very awesome pie chart called the "Discipleship Wheel," broken into eight different parts, to distribute to all of them.

I used a computer. I was proud. It was very professional looking.

"See, guys, just remember to do this stuff: attend worship, do short-term missions, pray, evangelize, give your money to the church and the poor, study the Bible, be a part of youth group, and . . ."

I can't remember what the other thing was. Something super-important.

". . . and then you can know you're doing all right with God."
Mike said, "Thanks!"

I saw Mike—he's now an engineer and a father of six—not long ago, and I told him how sorry I was, and we had a good laugh. Thankfully, he now has a better picture of just how good God is.

He now knows that God did not call us into Pie-Chart Life, however smart-looking the chart. God wants to know us.

He wants to know us, and He wants us to know Him. He wants us to want Him. Not ideas or abstractions about Him, but Him. Ultimately, this is a more restful life. Not just because it might mean some quiet, meditative moments—though they're wonderful—but because when we surrender control, there's so much less at stake in life for us.

We have nothing to prove, and when we really believe that, we'll hardly be quick to anger.

We have nothing to prove, and when we really believe that, we'll hardly be quick to anger. When we do get angry, we'll rid ourselves of the anger more easily. Remember: *Anger and rest are always at odds. You can't have both at once.*

We're told, in Psalm 46:10, to "be still," or to "cease striving" (NASB), and know that He is God. Some people are familiar with this verse but not the larger context, which is that of someone looking over the remains of a battlefield. The original Hebrew is suggestive of stopping the fight, letting go, and relaxing.

God wants us to drop our arms.

No more defensiveness. No more taking things personally. He'll handle it. Really.

Trust Him. Rest.

Quit thinking it's up to you to police people, and that God needs you to "take a stand."

God "needs" nothing.

Quit trying to parent the whole world. Quit offering advice when exactly zero people asked for it. Quit being shocked when people don't share your morality. Quit serving as judge and jury, in your own mind, of that person who just cut you off in traffic. Quit thinking you need to "discern" what others' motives are. And quit rehearsing in your mind what that other person did to you.

It's all so exhausting.

It reminds me of Aibileen's scene with Hilly in the movie *The Help*. Hilly is a judgmental, racist, conniving busybody full of religiosity and anger. Aibileen is her friend Elizabeth's hired help, and a wise woman who, when she finally confronts Hilly, is bracingly honest but still, somehow, loving:

"Ain't you tired, Miss Hilly? Ain't you tired?"[1]

It's a riveting and well-known scene. I don't think it's purely for the convincing acting (though, in my opinion, Viola Davis should've won an Oscar on the strength of this scene alone). I think it strikes a deeper chord. And it resonates with me, and even hurts, because Aibileen's words are piercing and fitting, and I feel that they were meant for me.

I've tried appraising people, determining their value based on how they treat me.

I've tried holding on to anger, harboring resentment, and doing the necessary mental gymnastics to justify myself, even if only in the court of my own opinion.

I've tried evaluating everything everyone else says, sifting through it to find if there's some way I've been slighted.

I've tried resisting God's clear command to forgive as He has forgiven me, and I've gone to the great effort to explain—again, if only to myself—how whatever I've done really isn't as bad as what that other person is doing to me.

It's really hard. It's really time-consuming. It's really a drain mentally, spiritually, and even physically.

This gavel, the one I awarded myself—who knows why?—is really, really heavy. I can keep pronouncing everyone else guilty for the rest of my life, but I'm not sure why.

I don't want this anymore. Maybe you know what I mean. So let me ask you . . .

Ain't you tired?

9

REVEREND OF THE DUMPSTER

There once was a pastor, in the days before the Internet took off, who availed himself of adult magazines when his wife wasn't around. He knew what he was doing wasn't right, of course, but he did it anyway.

His wife left for a few days on a trip, and once she was gone from their apartment, he brought his magazines out of hiding. Later, he was so frustrated with himself and his continuing addiction that he decided, once and for all, to throw the magazines away.

So he did. He took loads of them to the Dumpster, which sat at the base of their apartment's stairwell, and got rid of them.

Sadly—and perhaps you can relate to this—he later wanted them back. His wife was to arrive soon, and the trash hadn't been collected, so he returned quickly to the Dumpster. Struggling, he leaned over the side to reach the magazines, lost his balance, and fell inside, breaking his arm.

He couldn't get out.

It was just him. A pastor, trapped with his magazines . . . bleating for help in a Dumpster.

And that's where his wife found him.

Since hearing that true story, I think about that guy sometimes. But honestly, I don't think about what a loser he is, or what a hypocrite he is. Instead, I wonder if he's still married. I wonder if his wife forgave him. I think about what it might have been like to be so obviously busted, so humiliatingly, crushingly, can't-explain-this-one busted . . . and then forgiven.

And—you knew I was going here—*that's all of us*, if we're honest. It may not be pornography we're talking about, but in one way or another, we're all the Dumpster Pastor. I've found myself wondering what it would be like to be part of a church of nothing *but* Dumpster Pastors, people who know they've been caught, their lies exposed, and then set free. I think it would be a very, very fun, free, joyous church.

Walk into many AA meetings or Celebrate Recovery groups, and you'll find something like it. You can't join Alcoholics Anonymous and pretend you've got everything under control. When you join, you're saying, "I can't pretend anymore," and you're joining with people who are right there with you. There's something wonderful about that.

Also wonderful: If you're in an AA meeting, no one can walk in and yell, "Aha! I've got you! You're all hypocrites. You see, I know about you, and I'm going to go ahead and say it: *you are all alcoholics!*"

There would be a pause, some laughter, and maybe an invitation to sit down and join them.

There's a lot less stress when you've been found out.

There's a lot less stress when you've been found out. Pretending doesn't come so easily. You can't convince yourself that you're not just as guilty as everyone else anymore. You know the truth, and the truth has a way of setting you free.

And that includes a freedom from anger.

● ● ●

I think Dumpster Church would be the opposite of an angry place. We don't get angry when *we've* just been let off the hook.

It's just conjecture, of course, but I'm guessing, if you were driving home after being forgiven of a capital crime, you're going to let people merge in your lane without yelling at them.

When you're living in the reality of the forgiveness you've been extended, you just don't get angry with others easily.

I suspect our sense of entitlement to anger is directly proportional to our perception of our own relative innocence. So when that illusion is blown up, irrevocably, publicly, in our faces, it's very, very difficult to be angry with someone else.

So yes, as believers in Jesus, remember we've all been exposed publicly for what we are. The depth of our brokenness, the extent of our betrayal, has not only been the subject of news; it's changed history.

When did this public exposure happen? Two thousand years ago, our ugliness was made public on a hill, when a man stripped of His clothing was spat upon, made fun of, abandoned, and executed.

It happened because of us, and it should have been us, but we were let off the hook. When I take that in, both the depth of my betrayal and knowing that my punishment is no longer hanging over my head, I'm downright joyful. I'm extremely grateful.

And, as we already noted, in the human heart, gratitude and anger simply cannot coexist. It's one or the other.

Paul, writing to the Romans, didn't mess around on this point. He talked about how godless some people are, how boastful and proud and disobedient and heartless they can be, and then said this to the Christians he was writing to:

> If you think you can judge others, you are wrong. When you judge them, you are really judging yourself guilty, because you do the same things they do. God judges those who do wrong things, and we know that his judging is right. You judge those who do wrong, but you do wrong yourselves. Do you think you will be able to escape the judgment of God? (Rom. 2:1–3 NCV)

Yep, they were just as guilty. We're just as guilty.

I love how fair Jesus is on this, how He levels the playing field, so no one can honestly pretend he or she is righteous anymore. People want to say, for instance, "Well, I'm not an adulterer. I've never had sex with someone outside of marriage." But then Jesus comes along, in the Sermon on the Mount, and says if you've ever lusted after someone, you're just as guilty.

It makes brilliant sense too: just because you haven't had the *opportunity* to follow through on what you'd like to do, you're not morally superior to someone who *has* had that opportunity. You say you haven't murdered anyone? Jesus says you're just as guilty if you've truly hated someone. You just didn't have the guts to do what was in your heart.

Fair enough. On one level, of course, I don't like it, because it puts me on the same plane as a murderer, but, as I say, He's brilliant. He leaves us sputtering. Make no mistake: we're busted, at the bottom of the Dumpster.

And then He goes and dies for us.

● ● ●

Of course, as I keep making the point that we are not entitled to our anger, because we are just as guilty, that will sound extreme to some. Problem is, according to Jesus, it's actually not extreme enough.

In Matthew 18 He tells the story of the unmerciful servant, a guy who owes the king millions of dollars. The king orders him to be sold, along with his wife and kids and everything he owns, to pay back the debt.

The guy pleads with the king, and the king has pity and lets him go.

And then, remarkably, the same guy *won't* forgive someone else who owes *him* money. And—this is important—it's a small amount of money too. But the original servant, who'd been forgiven so much, won't forgive in turn.

This ticks the king off. Big mistake. Jesus concludes the story with the unmerciful servant getting tortured until he pays his original debts.

Gulp.

And this story is in direct response to a question about forgiveness. Peter had asked Jesus how many times to forgive, as in "How far do we go with this forgiveness thing? Seven times?"

Jesus says, effectively, "Not even close," and then lets us know that, before God, we are in far deeper debt than anyone needing forgiveness from us. In that story, we're not "just as guilty" as the one whom we need to forgive.

We're worse.

●　●　●

If I get to determine whether my anger is righteous or not, I'm in trouble. So are you. The reason: we can't trust ourselves.

"Trust in yourself" sounds like a perfectly normal thing to do. Problem is, for the believer, it isn't biblical at all. We are deceptive to the core:

> The heart is deceitful above all things, and desperately sick; who can understand it? (Jer. 17:9 ESV)

Or try this:

> There is a way that seems right to a man, but its end is the way to death. (Prov. 14:12 ESV)

That's a far cry from "trust in yourself," as is this:

> Trust in the LORD with all your heart, and lean not on your own understanding; in all your ways acknowledge Him, and

He shall direct your paths. Do not be wise in your own eyes;
fear the LORD and depart from evil. (Prov. 3:5–7 NKJV)

We struggle with trusting God to mete out justice. We're
afraid He *won't* mete out justice, that people won't get what they
deserve. So perhaps our entitlement to anger is our little way of
making sure some measure of "justice" is served.

We are too good at deceiving ourselves to know if we have
"righteous anger" or not. Maybe this is why there is no such
allowance in Scripture. Even so, we can fool ourselves into
thinking we're innocent, or justified, or victimized.

This human trait goes way back. Study Adam and Eve and their inter-
actions with God right after they disobeyed Him. Adam's very first
reaction was to blame Eve. Eve's very first reaction was to blame the ser-
pent. Victims.

> We are too good at deceiving ourselves to know if we have "righteous anger" or not. Maybe this is why there is no such allowance in Scripture.

Just watch football fans. One team's fandom is positive their receiver was inbounds when he made the catch, and
the other team's fans are truly convinced he wasn't. Same play,
same evidence . . . and half the fans will feel they've truly been
victimized by the ref's call.

Yes, we're absolute masters at changing reality to fit our
narrative.

But Jesus wants to disrupt all of this.

He did it with the men who were ready to stone an adul-
teress to death. They genuinely believed, no doubt, they were
doing the "right" thing. They were carrying out God's justice,

they thought. They were angry for all the right reasons. She was guilty, after all.

Then Jesus made it simple: *You can't do this, because you're all just as guilty. Every single one of you.*

Anger makes me think I have a right to hold the stone. I may not throw it, but I'll hold on to it, since the other person really did do that horrible thing. But in the story, all the Pharisees drop their stones. The "good" guys, the aggrieved defenders of the faith, walk away empty-handed. They've got nothing.

Jesus flipped their story upside down. And since He wants to do this for all of us, I say we let Him. When you do, you'll find you have no standing to hold on to anger, ever.

You're not going to like this, but face it for what it is, and say it out loud: "That person I'm angry with? *I'm worse.*"

It hurts, and we can reject that idea if we want. But at least we're engaging what Jesus actually *said*, what He actually tells us about ourselves in the "Unmerciful Servant" story, rather than devising a less radical, less demanding God of our own choosing.

Truth is, we want Jesus to leave our self-righteousness intact.

He wants to smash it.

10

IDEA: LET'S PUNCH BRANT IN THE FACE

Maybe you know the feeling: Everyone's doing something you know is wrong, something you find so offensive, but you don't know how to convince them of just how wrong it is. You *desperately* need to let them know how wrong they are, and how right you are, and you need a means to make a convincing, well-thought-out, thought-provoking, logical argument.

But how? How can you do this? How can you properly impart your sweeping message of disapproval?

It's obvious: get an awesome T-shirt. I got one that said Smoking Stinks.

I had one of these as a kid. It had a picture of a cigarette with smoke coming out of it, and Smoking Stinks was written in cursive, which made it even fancier.

Most people in our little Illinois town smoked. But as a

Christian, I knew smoking was evil, so it was great to finally have a T-shirt that so succinctly communicated my disapproval.

Look, it's simple, folks: You smoke? You stink. I don't smoke. I don't stink.

I win. Questions?

Now, *what*, exactly, do I win? Nothing, as it turns out. But I was a kid, so I have to cut myself some slack. I was just doing what immature humans do, and that is thinking it's my job to put people in their place. I also thought it was my job to single-handedly "win souls for Christ," and when these souls saw my impressive purity and how I abstained from worldly things, like cigarettes, they'd say something like, "Wow! I want to be like you. Tell me about this 'Jesus' who claimed to be the Jewish Messiah, the fulfillment of all prophecy, the hinge in the history of the universe, and who has inspired you to wear this Smoking Stinks T-shirt."

Just for the record: to date, exactly zero people have said that. But it's not too late.

● ● ●

Quick quiz! And this is a risky one, at least for me. I'm going to tell you a few things about myself, and then I'll ask you a question at the end. So be ready for the question.

Unless you're a PK (preacher's kid) like me, all of these statements are likely true:

Over the course of my life, I, Brant Hansen, have likely
    cussed far less than you.
I probably exercise far more than you.

I am likely far more "discerning" and conservative with my
family's entertainment choices than you are.

I've probably been drunk less than you. (Zero times, total,
in my life.)

I've likely done drugs less than you. (Again, zero times.)

I've possibly done more to help the poor than you.

I've probably been less promiscuous than you. (I was a
virgin when I got married and have never cheated.)

I've likely smoked less than you. And worn more
antismoking shirts.

I probably have less debt than you, since I'm debt-free.

I likely give away more of my money, and a higher
percentage, than you do.

I probably have less body fat than you, because I'm far more
disciplined about eating good food than you are.

I've likely baptized more people than you have.

And now, here's the question, so be honest: *How do you like
me now?*

A) I'm incredibly impressed, Brant. You're amazing. I want to
hang out with someone as inspiringly clean-living as you.

B) Maybe you mean well, but I'd kinda like to punch you in
the face.

C) There is no "kinda." I want to punch you in the face.

D) Seriously, Brant, I'm coming to punch you in the face.

Personally, I choose (C) because I want to punch myself in the
face. Hard.

Perhaps I'm wrong on this, but I doubt people will love God

more because of my list of moral accomplishments. They're more likely to be annoyed, and I don't blame them. Even worse, at least one person would probably think, *Yep, Brant's morally better than me. I'm a loser, just like I figured.*

Great. You lost. What do I win?

Truth is—and this goes for secular "righteousness," too, like bragging about buying your own carbon offsets, or your sanctimonious bumper sticker—precious few people are attracted to displays of moral fastidiousness. As an example, I just saw an article about the "10 Most Annoying Gwyneth Paltrow Quotes of All Time," all her own comments about how wonderfully pure her diet is. No one wants to hear that.[1]

> **Perhaps I'm wrong on this, but I doubt people will love God more because of my list of moral accomplishments. They're more likely to be annoyed.**

People are put off because our deepest, most heartfelt questions aren't, "Is Brant a really pure person?" or, "Can Gwyneth somehow, some way, maintain her flat abs with the assistance of an entire team of chefs and fitness professionals?"

That's not what speaks to us. That's not our question. What we're really wondering, what everyone's really wondering, is simply this:

Does God really, truly, after all I've done . . . love me?

●　●　●

Not long ago, I stole about six hundred dollars' worth of stuff from a friend. He was a "friendly colleague," to be more accurate, a fellow radio professional who published a daily "show prep" site. I knew him because we worked in the same town. I was a talk-radio host who was well known for being a follower of Jesus. He was a successful host at a country station, in addition to running his Internet business.

He invited me to lunch one day, along with the other people on his show, and we enjoyed talking. He told me he respected me as a radio pro, and the high regard was mutual. He wasn't particularly into the "Jesus thing," but was very respectful of my beliefs. Soon after, I moved to Florida to work in Christian radio, and he sent me an e-mail, sad that I was leaving but wishing me well.

Radio people, especially morning shows, pay about fifty dollars a month to get fresh ideas, to read takes on current events, or to find out what happened on TV last night so they can talk about it and seem up-to-date. Not long after starting on my new morning show in Florida, someone gave me a password to a show prep site, one of the best sites in the industry. It was my friend's site.

I used the borrowed password for about a year. I felt guilty about it at first, but as I tend to do, I rationalized it. I didn't have the fifty dollars a month, and besides, it wasn't as if it was costing him anything if I used his material. Over time, I didn't even think about it. I just downloaded and printed out his daily report to use on my show.

Until, that is, one morning, as I printed it out, and, for whatever reason, I suddenly felt another pang of guilt. It was during a show, about seven in the morning, when I sent it to the printer, and wondered, *Is it possible that he could know I'm downloading this? That he could know I'm in West Palm Beach, and see the IP address of people who are accessing his info, and just suspect it's me?*

As I was thinking that—not kidding, here—an e-mail pinged

into my box, *from him*. The subject line read simply, "What's going on?" I felt sick.

He did know. He knew I was ripping him off. I was the Christian broadcaster he actually respected, and I was pirating his stuff.

I could barely get through the show. I didn't have anything to say on the air, nothing funny, nothing at all. I didn't know how I was to handle this, but I knew I had to call him and apologize. I owed him six hundred dollars, and money was tight. I thought about having to explain that to my wife, when we had almost nothing in the bank.

So I stared at the phone for a while, and then I called him. I told him I was so sorry. And I told him I knew the irony of Christian Broadcaster Guy stealing from Secular Broadcaster Guy, and how I was embarrassed and at his mercy. I would pay him his six hundred dollars immediately.

He was amazingly graceful. He said we've all done things that we're embarrassed about. He told me he accepted my apology, and I should forget about it, and that he still respected me. (By the way, he told me that he hadn't known I was stealing his stuff; he just e-mailed to tell me he missed hearing me on the radio.)

He forgave me.

Truth is, while my sin is embarrassing, he's a smart guy, and he already knew I was a sinner. In fact, everyone who knows me does, even if I've never personally stolen anything from them. If I think I can put one over on people and convince them that I've got my act together, the only one I'm fooling is me.

And the same goes with you. If you think people are drawn to you by an impressive religious résumé, you're in for a shock. When people are in crisis or need to know that God loves them, that they're not alone, they don't seek out the guy who thinks he's Mr. Answer or who radiates superiority and disapproval. They want someone who loves God and who loves them.

Refusing to be offended by others is a powerful door-opener to actual relationships. I don't expect people who aren't believers to act like followers of Jesus. Why should they? How about I give up the sanctimonious act and just love them, without thinking I need to change their moral behavior?

Refusing to be offended by others is a powerful door-opener to actual relationships.

Why not leave that to God? He's still changing my own behavior, after all. Again, it's simple humility. I know God wants my heart and wants their hearts. He wants us to turn away from ourselves and turn to Him. He can handle the rest. He loves them even more than I do.

At some level, of course, I enjoy trying to control the behavior of others.

Only problem: I can't even fully control *me*.

11

ATHEISTS, SOCIALISTS, AND TOAST

I used to think that to be Christlike meant to be alienated and put off by the sin of others. But it's quite the opposite. *Refusing to be alienated and put off by the sin of others is what allows me to be Christlike.*

Recently, I saw an article in a mainstream online magazine about the hip-hop artist Lecrae, who's an outspoken believer. Lecrae loads his music with thoughtful reflections on all aspects of life, including—and especially—the good news of God's love for us. The article read:

"Christians have no idea how to deal with art," Lecrae said more recently, during a September speech to Christian leaders. "They say, 'Hey Lecrae you can't do that. That's bad. That's secular. You can't touch that. Hey Lecrae, your engineer is not a Christian. He can't mix your stuff. He's going to get sinner cooties on it.'"

"This is real. I wish I was making this up," he said.

Yeah, me too. I wish he were making that up.

The writer of the article went on to explain this mind-set to a mainstream readership, and I think he nailed it.

> Evangelicals adopted an isolationist mindset for much of the 20th century. Non-Christians, the thinking went, carried sin like a virus, and the point of following Jesus was to remain as pure as possible. Christians established their own communities, educational institutions and music festivals, separate from the rest of the world.[1]

Again, I wish it weren't true, and not just of evangelical culture generally, but of myself specifically. I used to think it was not only prudent but my duty to be offended by others' sins. Somehow, I took the example of the King of kings, who wanted to be with us so much that He lowered Himself to be born in a barn full of animals and manure, and I thought it meant I was supposed to raise myself above and away from the messy lives of others.

I guess I thought I was always on defense, guarding myself against the contamination, as though my heart weren't already contaminated with my own self-regard.

Worse, perhaps, I think I bought in to the idea that God and the Enemy are equals, caught up in the classic melodrama of evenly matched good versus evil. It sounds about right, with God on one shoulder and Satan on the other, whispering into our ears, one telling us to be nice and the other telling us to be selfish. (I'm not sure where I got that idea, but it may have been the noted theologian Fred Flintstone.)

But the kingdom of God is not on defense.

I used to read, in Matthew 16, where Jesus was talking about the "gates of hell" coming against the church and how they would not prevail against it, and I'd think, *That's great! We can stand up to the worst attacks.* But that doesn't make any sense. Gates don't attack. I'm kind of a military history nerd, and I still missed this. This reference isn't defensive at all. It's about being on offense. What it actually sounds like is this: Jesus is sending His followers out to love others, and they can go anywhere, even through the gates of hell, to do it.

Love people where they are, and love them boldly.

And if you really want to go crazy, *like* them too.

I have to throw in this caveat, or people will use it to miss the whole point: yes, it's true, if you are weak in a particular area, you are wise to set up boundaries in that area. Someone who is addicted to alcohol may wisely decide not to go to a bar. But let's stop aspiring to be "weaker brothers," or letting outlier scenarios give us an "out" from venturing into people's lives. Love people where they are, and love them boldly.

And if you really want to go crazy, *like* them too.

I love what author Mike Yaconelli once wrote: "Christians do not condone unbiblical living; we redeem it."[2]

In the book *Messy Spirituality*, Yaconelli told a story about a small group of American soldiers during World War II who sought out a burial site for one of their fallen friends. They were pulling out the next day, and were hoping to bury him in a fenced churchyard cemetery nearby.

As the sun was setting, they approached the house next to the church and knocked on the door. The priest answered. They asked him if they could bury their friend in the cemetery.

"I'm sorry," he replied, "but that's only for members of our church."

The priest went on to tell the soldiers they could, if they chose, bury their comrade near the cemetery but on the other side of the fence. They were saddened but had few options, so that's what they did.

The next day, they wanted to visit their fellow soldier's grave site one last time before moving on. When they came to the churchyard, they were shocked: they couldn't find his grave.

It simply wasn't there.

One of them went to the parsonage door and knocked.

"What happened to the grave we dug?" one soldier asked when the priest answered. "It's not there. We did it last night, and it's not there."

"It's still there."

The soldier was baffled.

"You see, last night, I couldn't sleep," the priest confessed. "All I could think about was what I'd told you, that you couldn't bury your friend inside our fence. I regretted that. So, last night, I got up—and I moved the fence."[3]

● ● ●

I now want to be that guy who moves fences. I want to be the guy who says, "Yes, I see the mess you've made of things, just as I have. But God wants us, mess and all. No matter what."

And the good news, too, isn't that God is disinterested in

what we do, that He doesn't care how we behave, or what we do to ourselves or others. It's good news that He *does* care about those things.

So He's going to change us, and if we want the status quo, we don't want Him. But that's not a guilt trip. His desire to change us is just further evidence that we matter to Him, and He loves us.

My goal with relationships is no longer to try to change people. It's to introduce people to a God who is already reaching toward them, right where they are.

This changes everything. It means everyone is welcome, and not just theoretically, but really: everyone—no matter what their political or religious beliefs—is welcome in my home, at my table.

I happen to be a pro-life, limited-government Jesus-follower. So you're an atheist and a socialist who's pro-choice and thinks Jesus is for losers? Fascinating! Say, how do you like your toast? Tell me more about your thoughts about Jesus and losers . . .

Refusing to be angry about others' views isn't conflict avoidance or happy-talk. It's the very nature of serving people.

Welcoming people into our lives isn't "glossing over important issues." Refusing to be angry about others' views isn't conflict avoidance or happy-talk. It's the very nature of serving people. I don't pretend the differences aren't there; I just appreciate that God has a different timetable with everyone.

And yes, I've seen wonderful things happen as a result of this newfound patience with people, things like great conversations and changed lives. But that's not even the point for me, because

I'm not responsible for changing people's lives. I'm responsible for faithfully loving them. As a believer, that means pointing them to a God who dearly wants them, and for whom I happen to know they yearn.

I don't control anyone, because that's God's job. That's His deal. I can just enjoy and love people. As I keep saying, I wish I would've known this sooner. I wish I could've seen the entire redemptive, narrative arc of the Bible, rather than cherry-picking a few bits that seemed, when isolated, to suggest disengagement with sinners. But the good thing is, I've finally learned:

Don't condemn the culture; redeem it.

12

ANGER'S FUN—
EXCEPT FOR THE
BOILING, BLAZING,
AND BURNING PART

So, overall, how does Scripture, which is well acquainted with injustice, describe anger?[1]

Well, anger is described as "fierce" and "cruel" in Genesis 49:7. It's "burning" in Exodus 11:8. In the same book, it's also described as a "blazing fury," and if you're not careful, it can "blaze against you" (Ex. 15:7; 22:24).

In Leviticus 26, anger is something given "full vent" and equated with "hostility" (v. 28). In Deuteronomy 7, it is associated with the words "burn" and "destroy" (v. 4). In 1 Samuel 20, we see an anger that "boil[s] with rage" (v. 30). Anger "will not be quenched," according to 2 Kings 22:17. In 2 Samuel 6, it bursts out (v. 8); in Job 4, it blasts (v. 9); and in Job 16, God Himself, in anger, "tears" and "pierces" (v. 9).

Anger is terrifying and fierce in Psalm 2:5. It's burning and consuming in Psalm 69:24, then smoldering intensely in Psalm 74.

In Isaiah 9:12, it's associated with a fist poised to strike. In chapter 30, it's demonstrated with flames, cloudbursts, thunderstorms, and hailstones (v. 30). In Isaiah 63:3, it tramples.

It doesn't exactly chill out in Lamentations. The words "engulfed" and "slaughtered" are used in chapter 3 (v. 43).

I'm not cherry-picking. There just aren't lots of references to anger in the Bible as something wonderful. And yet we're now told it's a "gift," for our use when we feel it's "reasonable."

We're also told we should be aroused to anger when we see one of God's commands being broken. Really? Then we're going to be busy . . . really, really busy. We're also going to be really, really angry, all the time—and that's just at *ourselves*, for starters.

Maybe I'm supposed to be angry that often, and maybe it's really a gift. Maybe it'll make my life more joyful and peaceful . . . so long as I don't also mind the burning, blazing, cloud-bursting, striking, thundering, hailing, tearing, piercing, trampling, slaughtering, boiling, and the occasional blasting.

If this is, in fact, what we're supposed to do—experience "righteous anger" whenever we're made aware of one of God's commands being broken—we'll be precisely what the world doesn't need and largely believes we already are: a bunch of uptight, seething hypocrites.

The Bible directs us to get rid of anger (Eph. 4:31; Col. 3:8), but the idea of "righteous anger" turns that directive on its head:

we can actually pat ourselves on the back for being offended and embracing anger.

And all that boiling, piercing, corrosive power becomes part of our lives—and destroys us.

● ● ●

When our son, Justice, was tiny, he was obsessed with one thing. Only one: he was completely smitten with *garbage*.

Yep, literal garbage. That's all he wanted, all he thought about. He loved trash. He would excitedly point out Dumpsters to us whenever we were driving about.

Trash. That's it. Nothing else.

We even got him a trash video. It was a full hour of trucks moving garbage around at the dump in big piles. He was mesmerized. No plot, no dialogue; just a lot of beeping from trucks backing up. Who knew there was a market for this?

We had hardwood floors, and I remember my wife and I were in the living room, and we heard a dragging sound . . . and there was Justice, beaming, dragging a bag of trash into the room. His love of garbage was inspiring.

It dawned on me that I could make him an offer. I could stand in front of him and offer him a crisp one-hundred-dollar bill for his bag of garbage. I could tell him, "Look, this is *way* more valuable. Just give me your trash, and I'll give you this hundred-dollar bill! Just hand it over! Give me your garbage . . ."

There's no way he'd do it.

And you know what? You and I are just like him.

We cling to our self-righteousness and can't possibly imagine giving it up. We think it's how we're supposed to live. *Wait: We're supposed to surrender the idea that we know others' motivations? We're supposed to give up thinking we know everyone's spiritual temperature? We're supposed to live without constantly assessing where we, ourselves, stand spiritually?*

We can't even imagine the world could look that way. This is our way of life. Honestly, we're obsessed with self-righteousness, sick with it, all of us.

Wait: We're supposed to surrender the idea that we know others' motivations? But our Father is holding out another way of living, entirely. He's saying it's far more valuable. He knows. He made us. He knows we can live better this way. We'll be under less stress. We'll be able to live in the moment. We won't be constantly offended, perpetually nursing hurts. He's telling us to hand over the idea that we know things we don't about ourselves and others, and simply be humble.

I've found myself thinking—even if I don't say it out loud—that part of my job as a Christian is assessing where people stand. Therefore, if I didn't try to make this assessment about others, I wasn't taking Christianity seriously enough, or something. I don't know what I was thinking.

What a sweet, sweet relief to not have to do this.

I don't know where people really stand with God. If someone asks me, "Hey, is that athlete a good Christian guy? I've heard he is," I now admit, right here and right now, that I have no clue. How would I know?

"Hey, Brant, you love U2. Is Bono really a good Christian?"

I have no response for this. You know, I love some of the stuff he does. I'm a fan. But even if I lived next door to him and hung out every single day with the guy for fifty years, I wouldn't know what's in his heart. (Usually, by the way, I think this question really means, "Hey, Brant, do you think Bono is trying as hard as I am to be a good Christian?")

Jesus had to point out to seemingly upstanding religious leaders that some prostitutes are closer to the kingdom of God than they were. Would you or I have known that?

Let's be blunt: people are able to fool even their own spouses for a very long time. It's happened very recently, with a high-profile evangelical Christian leader. Turns out he'd been leading a double life for decades, and his wife was devastated and humiliated at the news.

I don't know, ultimately, where people stand. I know what they need and what I need. I know we need Jesus. That's it. Period. Everybody. All of us. All the time. More of Him. That's all I know.

If people don't really know Him, they need to know Him. And those who do know Him need to see Him all over again. I'm already a believer, but the kingdom of God is so shockingly opposite the way the rest of the world works that I need constant reminding of what it looks like and how good it is.

It's simple, honestly. You can quit trying to assess everyone; quit pretending you know where people stand; quit fooling yourself into thinking you know what others are thinking, what's in their hearts. Let's be humble and admit what we don't know. What we do know is this simple truth: everyone, pastors and prostitutes, needs more Jesus.

You can really live like this. I've tried it. It's a complete reversal from the way many of us live, but it's doable. If I can do it, things look good for you too. I'm so glad the judging business is

God's business. I can't handle it. Neither can you, really, even if you think you can.

Some people grow up in horrific conditions, see unspeakable things, suffer horrible abuse, act out as teenagers, wind up in prison early, and know no other life. Others are born into wonderful, nurturing, disciplined families, and are "nice" by their very nature. Still others have devastating brain injuries, and their personalities change dramatically in a moment. Many folks have been through things I'll never understand.

> So how do I assess the relative spiritual temperature of these people? How do I determine where they stand with God? Answer: I don't.

So how do I assess the relative spiritual temperature of these people? How do I determine where they stand with God?

Answer: I don't.

● ● ●

Last night, I talked with a new friend of mine who shared that he's always seemingly been angry. "I spend half of my life with anger," he said. "I've always lost a tremendous amount of sleep because of it."

As I sat at his kitchen table, with his two adorable toddler daughters running around us, he told me that because he's now in recovery from drug addiction, he's had to make amends with people with whom he's been angry. So he called a guy who once beat him up and told him he was forgiving him.

"The guy was amazed, but it really wasn't for him. It was for me," he said.

"And did you sleep soundly that night?"

He laughed. "Yes! Finally! It's amazing how that happens. And you know what? I've found that when I'm not angry, I can finally be in the moment with my wife and kids. Finally. I can just be here. I'm not thinking about what other people did to me."

God knows how we're wired. He tells us to forgive and to get rid of anger. People made in His image would do well to listen. It means everything, not just for us, but for those around us.

Like two sweet little girls, who can now have their daddy in full.

Life is better this way. It's better when we admit what we don't know, realize our own moral status before God, and give up our made-up Right to Be Offended.

We think we want a right to "righteous anger." It takes a tremendous amount of humility, an extraordinary "dying to self" to hand over this desire, this job, this obsession, to God. But He made us, and He knows how we operate best. He says to hand it over.

And He's promising something of value that no one else— and literally, no other religion—promises. He's promising a release from the constant evaluation, never-ending striving, and relentless assessment of where we, and everyone else, stand.

He's promising a better way of life. He's holding it out to us, saying, "Hand over the garbage," and He means it, because He loves us, and He has something better to offer.

He's offering *peace*.

13

THE BIG QUESTION: WHAT ABOUT INJUSTICE?

t's fair if you are presently thinking, *Wait! Are we not supposed to be angry at injustice? Are you crazy?*

We're not. But this does not make me crazy. The fact that I enjoy puppetry when no one else is looking? *That* makes me crazy. My daily habit of eating an entire loaf of burnt toast every morning for ten years? Yes, that qualifies me. Sure. You got me.

But this? No. It's not as insane sounding as you think.

Yes, it's unnatural, completely against our instincts, exceedingly radical, certainly unfashionable, counterintuitive, and in violation of conventional wisdom.

Yes to all that.

But so is "Love your enemy."

● ● ●

Let's dispense with one idea at the very start of this chapter: that *anger* and *action* are synonymous. Often, we confuse the two, thinking that if we're not angry about an unjust situation, we're simply accepting it. That's completely false.

And it's telling, I think, that the two are so frequently conflated. We've so justified anger that we can't imagine doing the right thing without it. Earlier, I quoted an online devotional that questioned whether we actually ever accomplish *anything* without anger. The stunning thing, as I've talked with people about this, is how common that idea is.

Anger and action are two very different things, and confusing the two actually hurts our efforts to set things right.

Check out Twitter sometime. You can see anger all over the place. People upset about this, and "taking a stand" on that. This isn't surprising.

Of course, we're all thankful for the right to speak our minds. But here's what's odd about this confusion when it comes to injustice, anger, and action: a recent study found that people who join causes online are not more apt to actually do something—they're *less* likely to take action.

According to research from the University of British Columbia, if you click "Like" on "Help the Poor Children of Wherever," you're actually less likely to give actual money to help the actual poor children of Wherever.[1] It's "slacktivism" in action. ("Inaction" is more accurate.)

Let's face it: we're positively in love with "taking stands" that cost us absolutely nothing. We even get to be fashionable in the process.

We get to think we're involved, doing something, and if we're angry, we get to say, "My anger is righteous anger." And since it's "righteous" anger, it stands to reason that we're actually *more* righteous than the people who aren't angry like we are!

The myth of "righteous anger" actually impedes the taking of action, because it lets us congratulate ourselves for a feeling, rather than for *doing* something. Meanwhile, someone else, someone who didn't tweet about it, didn't get the bumper sticker, and didn't click "Like" on the cause, is actually sacrificing his or her time and treasure to genuinely benefit the poor children of Wherever.

Anger and action are two very different things, and confusing the two actually hurts our efforts to set things right.

There's a book called *Who Really Cares* that's about this very thing. It turns out that the people who are often the most indignant voices in protest of injustice are the least likely to part with their own resources to do anything about it.[2]

So often it's true: one person is angry—but it's someone else who takes action.

Another unfortunate result, in my experience, of the confusion of anger and action is this: Men, in particular, learn to see anger as masculine. They tend to think being angry, and acting out angrily, is very much part of what it means to be a man. (I could cite a million academic sources on this, but I'm just going to assume you agree with me. Plus, if I get back on the Internet right now, I'm going to wind up looking at cat memes again, and I really need to focus.)

When talking about this with people, this idea that the Bible doesn't ever endorse human anger as a solution for injustice, I get this reaction, particularly from men: "But we've got to do something!"

Yes, agreed: *Do* something. Take action.

"But if we don't get angry, we won't do anything."

Really? *Why?*

So you can't just *do* the right thing, because it's the right thing? The Bible gives us ample commands to act, and never, ever, says to do it out of anger. Instead, we're to be motivated by something very different: love, and obedience born of love.

The Bible gives us ample commands to act, and never, ever, says to do it out of anger. In fact, Paul wrote in 1 Corinthians, it's the defining motivation. If we do something good, even, without love, we're just a bunch of noise (13:1).

Acting out of love, to show mercy, to correct injustices, to set things right . . . is beautiful. Love should be motivation enough to do the right thing. And not "love" as a fuzzy abstraction, but love as a gutsy, willful decision to seek the best for others.

What the world needs, I think you'll agree, is not a group of people patting themselves on the back for being angry. We need people who actually act to set things right.

● ● ●

Doesn't anger help sometimes? Well, sure, sometimes, in the short run, anger can bring about some good things. Of course. But that's not a credit to anger; that's how the world works. The same could be said of practically anything.

Gluttony, for example, provides jobs for people. It doesn't mean gluttony isn't disordered; it's just that I can see how some good things, short-term, can come from it. That said, I rarely hear anyone speak of "righteous gluttony."

Same thing with bitterness: I've talked with some NFL players about this, how bitterness is *the* drive for some athletes, pushing them to lift weights harder, hit harder, practice harder; and as a result, they make a living. Some short-term good things can come from bitterness. But simply saying that "good might come of it" does not make the "it" a righteous thing.

Someone might be motivated by anger to do something that is otherwise good. But a relationship with God is like other relationships; it's not a moral "Did you do that?" checklist. The condition of our hearts is not a side issue. *Why* we do what we do matters infinitely.

Again, in 1 Corinthians, Paul said, "Though I bestow all my goods to feed the poor . . . but have not love, it profits me nothing" (13:3 NKJV).

You can recognize injustice, stand up to it, even sacrifice your life fighting it. And you can do it without anger. In fact, you'll do it better. You won't be remembered as angry, but as convicted of what's right, and loving to the very end. This kind of love leaves an impression on one's enemies that anger simply never will.

● ● ●

I just read an article called "The Gift of Anger," about how Christians should see their anger, when justified, as a blessing.[3] And we're given a test in so many of these articles, which is essentially this: to ask ourselves, "Is our anger justified? If yes, it's justifiable anger."

Nice test. I see what you did there, test-maker people.

Another Christian piece I read today says Jesus' story about the unmerciful servant is an example of when we should harbor anger.[4] This is the very story we talked about in an earlier chapter, where God is angry at those of us who do not forgive others, when we ourselves are guilty too. The rationale is, "See, God gets angry in this story. That means we should too!" But that's not the meaning of the story at all. We are not the king in that story. The king's anger does not give the unmerciful servant a valid basis for his own anger.

> In order for us to justify our right to anger, we have to confuse ourselves with God.

We are so protective of our own anger that we'll twist that story to justify it instead of rid ourselves of it. And it's instructive, given the way the unmerciful servant story is mishandled.

Think about it: *in order for us to justify our right to anger, we have to confuse ourselves with God.*

If we think the biblical writers didn't anticipate the level of injustice and brokenness in our modern world, we're being naive on an epic scale. Early Christians in many cases were being targeted, imprisoned, and killed. What's more, the Middle Eastern world was shot through with infanticide, slavery, racism, sexism, child abuse, unjust wars and occupations, torture . . . it's all there.

And yet, the early Christians got letters from their leaders telling them to get rid of anger, period. Even if you disagree with me, I think you'll find this is a fair question: *If our modern writers are accurate, and Christians really are called to anger against injustice, why is that call missing entirely from these letters?*

The early church dealt with injustice daily and was aware of widespread injustices affecting others. So why were they not told to get angry about it, if human anger toward true injustice is actually *righteous*?

Why isn't righteous anger ever listed among the things that a Spirit-filled life will bring us? If it's righteous, why is it not akin to the "fruit of the Spirit," like love, joy, peace, and gentleness? Why is anger in Scripture so consistently lumped in the *other* lists, with things like, say, slander and malice, with no exclusions for the "righteous" variety? (See, for example, Colossians 3:8.)

We aren't to just pretend anger away or feel guilty for the initial emotion of anger. But we are to deal with it, with the goal of eradicating it within us. This, of course, is not easy to do, but it's not complex to understand, either.

Dallas Willard, who's quoted at the beginning of this book, said we now have so many angry Christians simply because "they're not taught out of it."

Few ever present the radical implications of what it means to die to ourselves and what it means to practice a lifestyle of forgiveness. "Stepping out of anger," Willard says, "means you are surrendering your will to God. It means you have accepted that you don't have to have your way."[5] When I've read commentaries on Ephesians 4:31, where Paul says to get rid of bitterness, anger, evil speaking, and so on, the commenter very often inserts the word *unreasonable* before anger. But that's not in the text, and the commenter doesn't extend the "unreasonable" standard to anything else on the list. (What about "unreasonable bitterness"?)

"But didn't some biblical heroes act out of anger?" Well, sure they did. They were humans. I'm so thankful the Bible is not a just-so story, not a singsongy, children's pop-up book of

SuperClean Heroes. Its stories are of people, like us moderns, who lie and cheat and steal and harbor anger and occasionally even kill innocent people. It's a mess. To say, "Well, Moses got angry at injustice in Exodus 2" is not to say that we should kill Egyptians too.

Those stories aren't how-to templates for our lives; they're stories that point us, ultimately, to the goodness of God.

• • •

We've already mentioned Martin Luther King Jr. as a man who understood both the demand for justice and the myth of "righteous anger." Like any other human, and any other Christian, he found himself getting angry at being treated unfairly and seeing injustice at work. Anger is a natural response to feeling threatened.

But he knew he needed to get rid of his anger. During the famous bus boycott in Montgomery, Alabama, in 1955, King was blamed by the authorities for the lack of a settlement. He knew it wasn't fair. And he wrote this in his autobiography:

> That Monday I went home with a heavy heart. I was weighed down by a terrible sense of guilt, remembering that on two or three occasions I had allowed myself to become angry and indignant. I had spoken hastily and resentfully. Yet I knew that this was no way to solve a problem. "You must not harbor anger," I admonished myself. "You must be willing to suffer the anger of the opponent, and yet not return anger."[6]

For those who ask, "But how can we fight injustice without anger?" King's response is simple: *Be motivated by love.* Love for victims, love for bystanders, and even love for our enemies themselves.

> We are not advocating violence. We want to love our enemies.
> I want you to love our enemies. Be good to them. Love them
> and let them know that you love them.[7]

Does it matter if we're motivated by anger as long as we do something good with it in fighting injustice? For the Christian, it certainly does. Motives matter.

Dietrich Bonhoeffer, the German pastor and theologian, believed, too, that the idea of our own "righteous anger" is foreign to the Scriptures. In *The Cost of Discipleship*, he made it clear: "Jesus will not accept the common distinction between righteous indignation and unjustifiable anger. The disciple must be entirely innocent of anger, because anger is an offence against both God and his neighbour."[8]

So I may be crazy, but I'm not the only one. Throw me in with Bonhoeffer and King.

What's striking about Bonhoeffer is that he wasn't just a pastor and theologian, of course. He was an assassin. He was part of a bombing plot to kill Adolf Hitler. The plot ultimately failed—Hitler lived, while others died from the explosion—and Bonhoeffer was executed for his role.

Those who agreed with Bonhoeffer's earlier pacifism were appalled at his role in a killing. I can respect their position. But there are those, including me, who can understand why someone might survey a grave situation and make a considered, even sorrowful, choice to act on behalf of millions.

Action need not be born of anger, and I thank God there are

those who will act to defend the innocent simply because it's the right thing to do.

● ● ●

Feeling powerless is sometimes excruciating. We want justice, and we want it now. If we can't get it, we can at least harbor our self-righteous anger. Sometimes, it's all we think we can do.

The Bible tells us to do something truly revolutionary, certainly un-American, and completely at odds with that: *wait.*

> Wait on the LORD; be of good courage, and He shall strengthen your heart; wait, I say, on the LORD! (Ps. 27:14 NKJV)

> For evildoers shall be cut off; but those who wait on the LORD, they shall inherit the earth. (Ps. 37:9 NKJV)

> Wait on the LORD, and keep His way, and He shall exalt you to inherit the land; when the wicked are cut off, you shall see it. (Ps. 37:34 NKJV)

> Do not say, "I will recompense evil"; wait for the LORD, and He will save you. (Prov. 20:22 NKJV)

This is really, really, really, really, really hard. I know; I just wrote *really* five times, and that's pretty unprofessional, but I could've written a lot more. I know it's hard, because it's hard for me right now, and yet, there it is. *Wait!*

And if I'm overemphasizing by writing *really* a lot, the writers of the Bible emphasize *wait* far more. I picked just a few verses of dozens. Waiting is not a subtle theme of Scripture.

And yes, we're also told to be just and to love mercy, in the meantime: "The Lord has told you, human, what is good; He has told you what he wants from you: to do what is right to other people, love being kind to others, and live humbly, obeying your God" (Mic. 6:8 NCV).

Living "humbly" is the part I'm so often missing in my anger. I want comeuppance for the proud, and I want it now. I don't want to wait.

In fact, I don't fully trust God. I'm worried He won't handle things the way I'd like.

Worry and anger often go hand in hand. They're both about feeling threatened, and they both represent, ultimately, a lack of trust. But there's a flipside, and it's good news: we get to see all over again how freeing it really is to trust God.

My anger isn't a sign of trust; it's the very opposite. I'm worried someone's going to get away with something, like God's not noticing and it's all up to me. This kind of anger is perfectly human, of course, and perfectly natural, and just as perfectly destructive as any other kind of anger.

> Rest in the LORD, and wait patiently for Him; do not fret because of him who prospers in his way, because of the man who brings wicked schemes to pass. Cease from anger, and forsake wrath; do not fret—*it* only causes harm. (Ps. 37:7–8 NKJV)

So let's joyfully work for justice and mercy. And while we do it, let's trust that God, our Father, who actually loves us, and also loves mercy and justice more than we ever could, is ultimately going to set things right. We don't need to act like kids who've been abandoned and are forced to take matters into our own hands, defending ourselves at every turn. Our Father is coming home, and He tells us, over and over, He's going to take care of things.

Choosing to be unoffendable, or relinquishing my right to anger, does not mean accepting injustice. It means actively seeking justice, and loving mercy, while walking humbly with God.

And that means remembering I'm not Him.

What a relief.

THIS IS THE CHAPTER ABOUT HOW WE'RE JUST BARELY SMART ENOUGH TO BE STUPID

We humans are weird.

That's not just my editorial opinion. It's a biological fact.

We are remarkably unique among all the creatures on the planet. Other creatures feel threatened, just like we do. The big difference, though, is that when they feel threatened, it's because they're being chased by, say, a lion. And it makes sense that they're threatened, since a lion can kill them.

But humans don't need to be chased by a giant cat or wolves or a shark to feel threatened. We don't have to be chased by anybody, or anything. We humans are special, because we can manage to feel threatened while being chased by . . .

Absolutely nothing. And amazingly, *that "nothing" is killing us.*

Maybe you've had this scenario happen to you, the "near miss" in traffic. You're driving a car, and another car comes from out of nowhere, you both slam on the brakes, and you narrowly miss each other. You take a deep breath, say something like "Thank God," and then make sure everybody's okay.

But you also notice your whole body feels different. It's been flooded with hormones, specifically adrenaline and cortisol. Your body went into fight-or-flight mode, perceiving a threat. Your heart rate is now higher, and so is your blood pressure, in order to shoot energy into your body. You've got more sugar in your bloodstream now, too, thanks to the cortisol, and that can help your brain think under pressure.

What you may not be aware of is that when you're in this mode, the "oh-my-goodness-my-life-is-threatened" mode, your body actually automatically shuts down other functions. Your digestive system temporarily closes down, and so does your reproductive system, because you need neither to survive the moment. Your body wants to make you lighter so you can run away, so you may suddenly feel as if you need to go to the bathroom. That's how we're wired. It all makes sense. It's all to help us survive real threats.

All that stuff happens with animals, too, when they're being chased. If you're an antelope, and you're being chased by a pack of bloodthirsty hyenas, you're having this same thing happen, and maybe you're thinking, *This is awesome; my whole antelope body is making me run faster than I ever thought I could.*

I love the way I'm equipped with this very cool fight-or-flight response system.

Thing is, for the antelope, the whole thing is over pretty quick. I mean, he either gets away from the hyenas or he doesn't. In either case, the whole physiological reaction is short-lived. Just a quick blast, really. That's what fight-or-flight is for.

Robert Sapolsky is a neuroendocrinologist and primatologist at Stanford University, and he studies the way stress affects animals and humans. He's written a terrific book called *Why Zebras Don't Get Ulcers*, which deals with this very issue and explains it much better than I can.[1]

Zebras have very real threats but don't get ulcers because that stress-response episode is here and gone in seconds. But we humans—we highly intelligent, top-of-the-food-chain, we-can-put-one-of-us-on-the-moon humans—*invent* things to make us feel threatened.

Antelopes don't do that. They don't lie awake at night, wondering if another antelope is going to make them transfer to another location or maybe fire them. That's us. We do that.

An antelope doesn't lose sleep worrying it might have run up credit-card charges that it can't pay off. We do.

An antelope doesn't toss and turn, worried that his baby antelope is going to get aced out of the top-tier antelope pre-school. No, that's us. That's a human thing. We're the brilliant ones who think that way.

We are capable of imagining threats and staying in a kind of constant, low-grade fight-or-flight mode. We're capable of feeling threatened all the time, by things that haven't even happened and may not ever happen.

We're so smart, we can trick our bodies into physiological breakdown for no good reason.

Sapolsky says it's remarkable what our emotions can do to us, physiologically, compared to other species:

> We've got the same building blocks, but we use them in ways that are unprecedented. And let me give you an example of that: Okay, so you've got two humans, and they're taking part in a human ritual. They're sitting there silently, making no eye contact. They're still. Except every now and then, one of them does nothing more taxing than lifting an arm and pushing a little piece of wood.
>
> And if it's the right wood, and the right chess grandmasters in a tournament, they are going through six to seven thousand calories a day, thinking, turning on a massive physiological stress response, simply with thought. And it does the same things to their bodies, as if they were baboons who just ripped open the stomach of their worst rival, and it's all with thought, memories, and emotions.[2]

The effects of our ability to feel threatened long-term are absolutely devastating. We simply weren't designed to handle this. And it's not just ulcers, either, that are the problem. When we're stressed out over the long haul, everything falls apart.

Your muscles start to suffer from the tension, so there's often neck and shoulder pain, for starters. And your immune system starts to fail. You get sick more, and if you're already sick, your symptoms get worse. Your stomach starts to rebel. You get gastroesophageal reflux, or irritable bowel syndrome, in addition to peptic ulcers. Stress can affect your fertility and your reproductive organs. It affects your lungs too. If you have asthma, stress can make that worse.

Of course, there's also your blood. When your body is dealing with stress long-term, you can develop high blood pressure, blood clots, or atherosclerosis. Coronary heart disease can set in, leading to heart attacks.

Your metabolism gets messed up. You may gain lots of weight, or even develop diabetes. It can even affect your skin, making psoriasis or acne worse.

As Sapolsky says, zebras don't have to deal with this. They don't dream up potential threats. They don't stay in perpetual fight-or-flight mode.

Sapolsky describes himself as a "strident atheist," so he's not trying to make a theological point with this. But it's fascinating that his conclusion, from his decades of research about threats, stress, and physiological response, is that we should not borrow trouble from tomorrow.

For the person who's familiar with the teachings of Jesus, that theme sure rings a bell. Here's Jesus, two thousand years ago:

> "Therefore I say to you, do not worry about your life, what you will eat or what you will drink; nor about your body, what you will put on. Is not life more than food and the body more than clothing? Look at the birds of the air, for they neither sow nor reap nor gather into barns; yet your heavenly Father feeds them. Are you not of more value than they?" (Matt. 6:25–26 NKJV)

Animals don't harm themselves with worry. They don't go into fight mode by creating threats with their imaginations. Humans do.

So Jesus says to take our lessons from the birds.

● ● ●

Jesus' next statement is worth looking at closely, in light of new research: "You cannot add any time to your life by worrying about it" (Matt. 6:27 NCV).

The research says that stress can even make our DNA appear older. Remarkable. Stress, the response to threat, is designed to equip us to live longer, and yet being anxious doesn't lengthen our lives at all. It ages us.

It shouldn't be surprising to me, I guess. But I'm struck again by the genius of Jesus and also the love of God. That He would talk to us in such a tender manner still makes me pause. He made us; He knows how we operate, and He watches us, alone among the creatures of the world, taxing our bodies by imagining threats and things that haven't happened.

We're silly little things.

Just as we've invented "righteous anger," we've justified our worry, our constant sense of threat and insecurity. But Timothy Keller tells us that worrying is, ultimately, simple arrogance: "Naturally, if you love people, you're going to worry about them. But do you know where constant worry comes from? It's rooted in an arrogance that assumes, I know the way my life has to go, and God's not getting it right. Real humility means to relax. Real humility means to laugh at yourself. Real humility means to be self-critical."[3]

We hold on to worry because we don't trust God. We hold on to anger because we don't trust God. We feel threatened because we're insecure, and we're insecure because—surprise!—we don't trust God.

When you start practicing it, you realize: choosing to be unoffendable means actually, for real, trusting God.

When you start practicing it, you realize: choosing to be unoffendable means actually, for real, trusting God.

The sooner we start this, the healthier we'll be. Not just now and not just physically, but long-term and spiritually. C. S. Lewis wrote about this lifetime trajectory, and how "little things" wind up shaping our entire existence, in *The Great Divorce*:

> Hell . . . begins with a grumbling mood, and yourself still distinct from it . . . Ye can repent, and come out of it again. But there may come a day when you can do that no longer. Then there will be no you left to criticize the mood, nor even to enjoy it, but just the grumble itself going on forever, like a machine.[4]

Choosing to be unoffendable and relinquishing our "right" to anger is a means of unplugging this machine before it gets going.

If security were based on reality, Hollywood stars would feel secure in their fame. They don't. Powerful politicians would feel secure in their power. They don't. And good-looking people would feel secure about their good looks.

Guess what?

"I am insecure," says Cameron Russell, supermodel. She

explains: "If you are ever wondering, 'If I have thinner thighs and shinier hair, will I be happier?' you just need to meet a group of models because they have the thinnest thighs and the shiniest hair and the coolest clothes and they're the most physically insecure people on the planet."[5]

The most physically insecure people on the planet, and therefore the people most easily threatened regarding their looks . . . are supermodels.

So what have we learned from this? If your security is based on your looks—or property or achievement, for that matter—you're in for a life of stress, because whatever it is you think you need, once you get it—if you ever get it—there's no guarantee you won't lose it.

Speaking of "security," I once met the Ultimate Dude.

I was in Afghanistan, working with the hospital network CURE International, and they assigned him as security to make sure I didn't get killed.

Let me describe his awesomeness: He can speak Dari, the local language, because he's smart. He's also six-foot-four and in perfect condition. He can handle weapons, because he's a Special Forces veteran. He's got combat experience.

He also looks like Jon Hamm and appears—no lie—twenty years younger than he is.

Did I mention he was smart? He's owned restaurants, apartment buildings, and several very successful medical businesses in the United States.

And he's an inventor, developing tactical wear for dozens of militaries and police forces worldwide.

So, yeah, he's impressive.

Oh, I forgot to mention: He's theologically astute. His dad was chairman of the board at one of the top seminaries in the United States.

And, oh yeah, he played big-time college football. He started on the defensive line for a Big 12 team. He does walk with a slight limp, but even that seeming vulnerability becomes impressive when you hear the story of how he hurt it jumping out of a helicopter on a mission.

So I'm already feeling inferior. But when we walked in CURE's hospital, the top plastic surgeon at the hospital—Afghanistan's top doc at healing children from disabilities—came running over to us, shouted the Ultimate Dude's name, and embraced him.

Why? Because the Ultimate Dude *taught him how to do the plastic surgeries at the hospital.* He's a surgeon too. One of the best. I neglected to mention that.

And by the way, when I met the Ultimate Dude, he was getting ready for his wedding. He was marrying a runner-up in the Miss Universe contest. Some of his celebrity friends would be there—like best-selling international-thriller authors who use him to help them shape stories.

I'm not making this guy up. He really exists, and I really like him. He's such a great guy and a huge blessing to people in many countries. CURE has healed so many children, done so much for the "least of these" (Matt. 25:40 NKJV), and the Ultimate Dude has been part of that. It's all amazing.

If I were that guy, I would have a hard time not just walking around thinking, *I'm so awesome I can barely stand it.*

So he's a Christian, and also a great-looking, tall, athletic, wealth-making, beauty-queen-marrying, Special Forces–serving, celebrity-befriending, weapons-bearing, multiple-language-speaking, business-starting, cutting-edge-equipment-inventing, world-hopping, child-saving plastic surgeon.

And there's one more thing . . .

He's insecure.

He told us as much. He really struggles with it. He feels as though he's trying to live up to something, and he doesn't know what, and he feels he's falling short. I'm so thankful for his honesty. (Though my first thought was actually, *Great. Now he's authentic and likable too?*)

But as he told us over dinner that it's just how he is, and he doesn't want to be this way, I believed him and respected him more when he admitted it. We can all relate.

But still . . . why? What could you possibly need to do besides all this?

"I don't know," he admits. "I really don't."

● ● ●

The lie, for most of us, is that we'll "get there," that we'll somehow, someday, make it to a point where that thing, that whatever, that we think we need to be secure, is finally ours, and we won't be threatened anymore, because we made it.

But there is no "there." It's such a pervasive lie, this notion that security comes from something besides God Himself, that professing Christians—even accomplished people in Christian culture—inhale it. Most of my friends who work in Christian radio would agree: there are many in our field, along with many

Christian musicians and authors and pastors and actors, who radiate insecurity.

For whatever reason, they're still pulling, chafing, and striving for the applause, and there's simply never, ever going to be enough of that.

We can put a Christian veneer on our striving, but it's insecurity nonetheless, made even uglier by our attempts to place it in a "ministry" context. That context often allows us to fool ourselves, and—once again—justify our selfish motives as "righteous."

We think some level of applause will satisfy us. We are delusional.

It may not be fame for you. But if you find your value— your "glory," as Scripture refers to your self-worth—in *anything* besides your identity as someone loved by God, you are never going to be truly content. That means ever-present threat, which makes being offended a way of life.

And that state of constant threat, that way of life, is deadly.

15

NOTHING LEFT TO LOSE

There's only one way to not be threatened by anything, and that's if you have nothing to lose.

And this is where this choosing-to-be-unoffendable business really becomes not only possible but also completely consonant with the teachings and life of Jesus. Just making the choice, and being mindful each day that "I'm not going to let people offend me," is very helpful, and it will make life better.

But ultimately, if I'm living in fear of losing something—whether it's security through status, looks, money, family, whatever—I'm going to be fearful, more easily threatened, and therefore prone to anger.

There's a song called "I Surrender All" that I remember singing as a kid in church. The lyrics are "All to Jesus I surrender / All to him I freely give."[1] I distinctly remember singing it once and hoping God wasn't listening. I actually didn't want Him snatching my favorite puppet, a green, furry monster named Burp.

No, not him. Not Burp, Lord. So yeah, I "surrender all," except for Burp . . . and my Hot Wheels, now that I think about it.

And then I heard stories about people losing their moms or their brothers or their entire families, and I thought, *God, I can't surrender that to You. I'm so sorry. I don't mean this song at all.*

I still struggle with that. I've got my own kids now. I can't even think about losing one of them. And yet, the song "I Surrender All" is surely appropriate: God wants us to give Him everything—even our children. Even our very lives.

A woman named Amy once e-mailed me about this. Here's what she said, and for what it's worth, my response:

Brant, my dog growled last night and I thought of this question and decided I'd ask you. My husband travels a lot (like 2 weeks a month) and so I am home alone with my two babies, my dog, and my two cats, and all the scary noises and shadows that make you wonder how safe you really are. I read a prayer book to my babies at night (just a collection of prayers) and a couple of them contain "Protect my family," "Watch over us," etc. . . . but here's my hiccup: God lets bad things (horrible things) happen to good people . . . to HIS people . . . People are raped and murdered every day, so how is trusting God to keep us safe supposed to happen?? Yeah, Daniel may have walked through a den of lions unscathed, but I'd be willing to bet Stephen felt every stone that was thrown at him. So how do we sleep at night knowing the world is full of evil and that sometimes (a lot of times) that evil hurts good people??

Amy

Amy,

Okay, here are my thoughts, such as they are. I think a *lot* of people are asking this question, even if they dare not ask it out loud.

As a dad, I think the answer to this is scary. And this may not be true for you; it may not be exactly your inner conversation, but the conversation can go something like this:

Honest question: *If I am a good Christian, and have faith and stuff, will God protect my children?*

Honest answer: He might. Or He might not.

Honest follow-up question: *So what good is He?*

I think the answer is that He's still good. But our safety, and the safety of our kids, isn't part of the deal. This is incredibly hard to accept on the American evangelical church scene, because we love families, and we love loving families, and we nearly associate godliness itself with cherishing family beyond any other earthly thing.

That someone would challenge this bond, the primacy of the family bond, is offensive. And yet . . .

Jesus did it. And it was even *more* offensive, then, in a culture that wasn't nearly so individualistic as ours. Everything was based on family: your reputation, your status—everything. And yet He challenges the idea that our attachment to family is so important, so noble, that it is synonymous with our love for Him.

Which leads to some other spare thoughts, like this: *we can make idols out of our families.*

Again, in a "Focus on the Family" subculture, it's hard to imagine how this could be. Families are good.

But idols aren't made of bad things. They used to be fashioned out of trees or stone, and those aren't bad, either. Idols aren't bad things; they're *good* things, made Ultimate.

We make things Ultimate when we see the true God as a route to these things, or a guarantor of them. It sounds like heresy, but it's not: the very safety of our family can become an idol.

God wants us to want Him for Him, not merely for what He can provide.

Here's another thought: As wonderful as "mother love" is, we have to make sure it doesn't become twisted. And it can. It can become a be-all, end-all, and the very focus of a woman's existence. C. S. Lewis writes that it's especially dangerous because it seems so very, very righteous. Who can possibly challenge a mother's love?

God can, and does, when it becomes an Ultimate. And it's more likely to become a disordered Ultimate than many other things, simply *because* it does seem so very righteous. Lewis says this happens with patriotism too.

Mother love, even when disordered and placed before a desire for God Himself, always looks perfectly justified. And that's why it's deadly.

Children are truly gifts from the Lord. But still it remains: God wants us to want Him for Him, not His gifts.

And this is the whole point of trust.

> **We say "I trust Jesus," or "Trust in the Lord, and . . ." and all that stuff. But here's where the words actually mean something: What if . . . the worst happens? Do you still trust Him?**

We say "I trust Jesus," or "Trust in the Lord, and . . ." and all that stuff. But here's where the words actually mean something: What if . . . the worst happens? Do you still trust Him? Do you believe it's really the end of the story if it does happen? Isn't that the point of trust itself, that you're stepping into mystery?

Job is the classic example. He had no idea what was going on, and he was left with only one thing: his trust in God Himself. He did not know the big picture, and yet he believed . . . *There has to be a picture, here, and it's one that I can't see.* As we know from the story, he was right. There was a backstory; he just didn't know what it was.

Do we *really* believe that God is good and will ultimately set things right? The real trust comes, I'm afraid, when what we think is "right" in our present reality doesn't happen.

Not long ago, my wife and I visited the mom and dad of a little girl who was the victim of an unspeakably horrible crime. A relative was in their home for Thanksgiving, and went on a shooting spree, concluding with deliberately taking the girl's life while she slept in her bed.

We sat in the little girl's room, days after the shooting. The dad sat on her bed and pulled down a beautiful, embroidered picture that was on the wall above it. He was crying, and pulled down the picture and showed the back of it to us.

He still thinks God is good. Somehow.

"I feel like we're only seeing this part right now, where it looks like chaos," he said. "But someday we'll see the front, where the stitches make more sense, and it will be beautiful. It doesn't make sense, but I have to trust God."

There are those who would say he's naive, but I think this is the very essence of trust, and the whole point of it.

We see dimly now, and we know in part now, but we will someday see it all. This is trust.

And one last, radical thought:

By becoming a Christian, we say we are giving our lives to Christ. If that's true—if we've given our lives to Christ—we've given it all. Everything.

And if that's true, it includes—and boy, is this tough to say as a dad—it includes our very children. They're His.

No one can take anything, or anyone, from His grip. They can take from ours, but not His.

So watch them sleep, and thank God for them, and know that they're on loan. He loves them even more than you do. And whatever happens, He's got the big picture; we don't.

That is trust.

Best,

Brant

16

AND HERE'S THE CHAPTER
I KEPT PUTTING OFF . . .

I knew this one was to be about the love of God, and I wanted to write it while on some kind of "spiritual high" so I could somehow write about it poetically, and it would just flow or something. I really did. That was the plan.

But that's not happening, apparently. I haven't felt particularly spiritual in a long time, and that's not out of the norm for me, for a lot of reasons. And now, I'm wiped out from a difficult week at work, and I'm particularly aware of my own sinfulness too. So I'm asking God to have mercy on me as I write this, and to help me anyway. Maybe it's for the best, since—I'm now convinced of this—most people who genuinely want to know God are not living in a persistent, perpetual state of amazement at His love.

And yet, His love is amazing. And His love *is* persistent and perpetual and unrelenting, even as our emotions, and our attention spans, aren't. The goodness of God is not dependent on my attentiveness to it. It does not come and go, wax and wane, or suddenly vanish like my misguided, untrustworthy emotions.

We're just not very attentive, honestly.

We're all a little bit like Dug the dog in the 2009 movie *Up*—kind of airheaded. We can sing "Amazing Grace" and be taken by it all, by the sweeping scope of God's love for all of us, His willingness to forgive us, and His desire to know us, and His unending—*Squirrel!*—and how He loves us in spite of our—*Seahawks game today!*—and "His grace will lead me . . ."—*I forgot to e-mail that guy*—"We've no less days to sing God's praise than when we've first begun" . . . *and I totally smell coffee; is someone making coffee?*

And you know what? God's grace is still amazing. We can ignore it, let it slide from our awareness, and yet . . . there it is.

Once, I forgot my keys in a church building, just as a group of us were getting ready to leave. Losing stuff is a lifestyle for me, so I was kind of proud that I remembered I'd left them down the hall and up the stairs, in the kitchen area.

It was dimly lit, but as I was gracefully running down the hallway, I saw a post in the middle. I avoided it deftly, and ran to the left side, before athletically darting up the stairs, grabbing the keys, crisply pivoting, bounding confidently back down the stairs, sprinting effortlessly down the hallway—and then smartly slamming my entire body into a plate-glass wall.

I shattered it. With my face.

Apparently, the other side of the post had glass from ceiling to floor. It was reinforced with wire mesh, so I didn't make it through. I just hit it, full sprint, and shook the entire building.

In the emergency room, I remember thinking, *You know, this is interesting. I was 100 percent sure there was nothing there. But there was, in fact, something there. I know this, because, among other observations, I note that I am bleeding profusely. Plus, my face hurts.*

I was completely convinced the hallway was clear. It's funny how reality didn't change to fit my interpretation of things. And by "funny," of course, I mean "only funny, like, ten years later."

Whether or not you currently feel that God is around doesn't alter reality. Whether or not you feel He loves you, or even that you are worthy of His love, doesn't change reality either.

Whether or not you currently feel that God is around doesn't alter reality.

What does this have to do with being unoffendable? Everything. That is, it changes everything if I'm attentive to it. It's the best news ever. Here's how Brennan Manning described the news:

> Because salvation is by grace through faith, I believe that among the countless number of people standing in front of the throne and in front of the Lamb, dressed in white robes and holding palms in their hands (see Revelation 7:9), I shall see the prostitute from the Kit-Kat Ranch in Carson City, Nevada, who tearfully told me that she could find no other employment to support her two-year-old son. I shall see the woman who had an abortion and is haunted by guilt and remorse but did the best she could faced with grueling alternatives; the businessman besieged with debt who sold his integrity in a series of desperate transactions; the insecure clergyman addicted to being liked, who never challenged his people from the pulpit and longed for unconditional love; the

sexually abused teen molested by his father and now selling his body on the street, who, as he falls asleep each night after his last "trick," whispers the name of the unknown God he learned about in Sunday school.

"But how?" we ask.

Then the voice says, "They have washed their robes and have made them white in the blood of the Lamb."

There they are. There *we* are—the multitude who so wanted to be faithful, who at times got defeated, soiled by life, and bested by trials, wearing the bloodied garments of life's tribulations, but through it all clung to faith.

My friends, if this is not good news to you, you have never understood the gospel of grace.[1]

As I said, the best news ever. God still loves us. He has not abandoned us. Every hope we've ever had—that someone would find value in us, would think we were worthy of love, would find us enjoyable and attractive and pleasing and worthwhile—is met in Him. God *Himself* loves us!

His love trumps everything. And nothing, Paul wrote in Romans, can separate us from that love.

Nothing.

And, he also wrote, if you put your trust in Jesus, there is no condemnation for you. None. You are off the hook. This is so stunning, so hard to actually believe, because nothing else in the world seems to work that way. *It's not based on my performance? It's based on what God has done for me? He loves me because . . . He just loves? It's who He is? He's not constantly evaluating my religious "goodness"? He's not angry with me? Seriously?*

It's a massive pressure relief. When I take it in, I'm still shocked. Really? I can see where a lot of those old hymn writers were coming from. "Amazing love, how can it be?"[2]

I'm a moral failure whose mind has drifted while even writing the last few paragraphs, with thoughts ranging from silly to immature to rebellious to lazy to selfish. I'm inconsistent to the core. But in a very real sense, it just doesn't matter. I want to grow up, but my Father loves me even as I am.

It's incredible news.

And that matters, when it comes to our offendability. Imagine you open your e-mail and there's actually some great news: someone wants to give you a hundred million dollars. (Now that I think about it, I get this offer from Nigerian friends on a daily basis. But say this is legit.) Chances are, after getting the money, you won't be quickly offended when someone cuts you off in traffic a few minutes later.

Better example, maybe: You've just been given the news by your doctor that your daughter's cancerous tumor, once thought to be terminal, is nowhere to be found. She's healed. You then notice you have a text message from that annoying guy at work, asking you to cover for him again. Are you angry?

The reality is this: The "good news" is, ultimately, even better. But you and I are forgetful people, and we get distracted, and we certainly don't always live in the reality of it. We need to be more attentive, and having people and disciplines in our lives to remind us of that great news will help us be remarkably slow to anger and offense.

●　●　●

But here's a bigger problem, and it's based on years of interacting with thousands of self-described Christians: It's not merely that we're not attentive to the fact that God loves us. *I suspect many of us actually just don't believe it.*

I suspect this because our behavior gives us away. After all, what we believe isn't what we say we believe; it's what we do. And what many of us do, as far as I can tell, is strive and strain and push and pull and work and worry and even anguish to try to somehow win favor with a Father who's already pleased with us. I could spend an hour on the radio, reciting scriptures about how we are now no longer under law, and how, if you've put your faith in Jesus, God has adopted you into His family, and I already know the inevitable response: Christians lined up to tell me it's not really quite true, that the real issue is that we need to stop sinning right now and work harder.

No wonder we get so angry. We're displeased with others because we're convinced God is displeased with us. We "believe" God loves us, but we suspect it's provisional, based on whether we ever get our act straightened out. That's a lot to carry.

If Christians are indeed the most easily offended people on the planet, this burden would go a long way toward explaining why. We're the ones convinced God has six hundred–plus rules—rules we know we can't keep—and that He's ticked off at us. But we try to keep them anyway. It's a prescription for immense frustration with ourselves.

And then we see other people not trying as hard as we are, and that's downright enraging. We hope God will give them their comeuppance someday, because if He doesn't, what the heck are we doing all this for?

So we believe the "good news," but not really. Not fully. We simultaneously do and we don't. Humans manage to do this with a lot of things. Many of us are a lot like the man in Mark 9, who begs Jesus to help his boy, who's being oppressed by a demonic spirit.

> When [the demon] saw [Jesus], immediately the spirit convulsed [the boy], and he fell on the ground and wallowed, foaming at the mouth.
>
> So [Jesus] asked his father, "How long has this been happening to him?"
>
> And he said, "From childhood. And often he has thrown him both into the fire and into the water to destroy him. But if You can do anything, have compassion on us and help us."
>
> Jesus said to him, "If you can believe, all things are possible to him who believes."
>
> Immediately the father of the child cried out and said with tears, "Lord, I believe; help my unbelief!" (vv. 20–24 NKJV)

I believe; help my unbelief! I just said that many of us are like this father, but maybe that's not true. Maybe we're not as honest as he was. So let's match his transparency before Jesus and admit we struggle with this.

And we can, because—get this!—Jesus didn't blast the guy. Instead, He made his dreams come true. There's no, "Are you kidding me? You *still* don't fully believe?"

Jesus set the boy free, and a father got his child back. No lectures, no diatribes.

By our standards, our ideas of rightness, it makes no sense. The way Jesus treats people often doesn't, by our reckoning. I mean, take this little test:

What does a properly religious leader do when seeing his so-called best friends for the first time after they disowned him and betrayed him in his hour of need?

A) Show them the error of their wicked ways by
   pronouncing harsh, deserved judgment upon them.
B) Give them a stern talking-to, but offer forgiveness if they
   prove themselves truly penitent.
C) Fry 'em up a hearty breakfast.

Jesus chose C.

And the breakfast didn't even come with a good scolding or an ironic, "Hey, nice job, fellas. Appreciate the way you handled that with such class." He just wanted to be with them again.

God walked among us. Even though we completely messed everything up, He took on flesh, lowering Himself to be with us, and walked in our world. He let us mock, bruise, and beat Him, and deliberately subject Him to an utterly humiliating capital punishment on display for all. He let us do that.

He wanted to be with us that bad.

And there He is, encountering His friends for the first time, and while they're coming back toward shore in their boat, God Himself is making breakfast.

You suspect you're unlovable? He loves you. You wonder, deep down, if anyone could really, truly know you and still want you? He knows you better than you know you. And He wants you.

You've given up on yourself? He hasn't given up on you. This isn't feel-good talk; it's the rightful conclusion we can draw from the cross itself.

He still loves us because He's a Father . . . the One we've always wanted.

WE'RE ALL WAITING FOR SOMETHING . . . THAT ALREADY HAPPENED

In Khaled Hosseini's magnificent book *And the Mountains Echoed*, one of the characters, Nabi, reflects in his later days on his life as a driver and butler in Kabul, Afghanistan, and the lives of those he's served. After a long recounting of pain, love, hardship, and hurt, Nabi says, "I suspect the truth is that we are waiting, all of us, against insurmountable odds, for something extraordinary to happen to us."[1]

That has a ring of truth about it. I've sometimes caught myself repeatedly checking my e-mail, for instance, with a vague sense of hope. I've had to ask myself, "What, exactly, am I hoping is going to pop up in my e-mail?" I'm not sure. But I'm hoping for something new, some good news, from someone. I want something extraordinary to happen.

I may be alone in this, but I don't think I am. We're all checking for some news, out of habit, even. We're mindlessly doing it, mechanically reaching for our phones, and hoping . . . for something.

Like Nabi, I think we're all waiting, all yearning, for something that will change everything. Something remarkable, indeed, that makes us, finally, amazingly significant and completely secure. We're waiting for something *extraordinary.*

My question is, what if that extraordinary thing has *already happened*?

What if we knew that the King wanted to be with us, wanted us in His family, His home . . . *forever*?

● ● ●

We modern Westerners have difficulty relating to the idea of a king. So I was struck when reading Laurence Bergreen's *Over the Edge of the World*, a book about the travels of Ferdinand Magellan and his crew, which lends clarity to the concept of "king" in so many cultures.

When they arrived in a Pacific island kingdom, they wanted an audience with the king. But they were told that no one could speak directly to him. If they wanted to say something, they had to tell a servant. And that servant would then have the honor of giving the message to another servant, one with a higher rank.

The high-ranking servant was allowed to speak to the brother of the governor. And the governor's brother was allowed to speak to a servant of the king. But not directly, of course. No, he could only speak through a "speaking-tube" that ran through a wall. The servant on the other end of the tube would then, and only then, relay the message to the king.[2]

The whole thing reminds me of working with my college's financial aid department back in the day, but that's not the point. The point is, Bergreen's description is true to the traditional idea of a king—an inaccessible, ordained-by-the-gods-if-not-a-god-himself king.

But the King of kings wants *you* so bad He'd give up His only Son to be with you?

He not only allows it, but *desires* that you and I—lowly us!—talk to Him often, whenever we want?

He's not asking us to try harder, but to *trust* that the work is already done to bring us into His family?

He wants to spend eternity—His eternity—with us?

Yes.

If we're mindful of this, and if we really believe it, how does this not leave us stunned and joyful? How does it not leave us less apt to take, and keep, offense? How can we continue to so easily feel slighted and hurt?

If we really believe it, we'll be known for being less apt to criticize, slower to anger, more forgiving. We'll be known for being loving toward one another, because we now have the resources to do just that. We've finally found what we've always wanted—significance and security, directly from the only One who can really give us both: the King of kings.

In fact, if this is true, that very love toward one another would be an accurate test of whether we really believed all this. If we loved others with a newfound patience, a refusal to take offense, and a lack of self-seeking, it would be evidence that all this is real.

The best evidence, maybe. Even better than apologetics

seminars or evolution/creation debates or even Christian T-shirts with "Jesus" substituted for the Reese's logo.

If this is all true, then our very refusal to be offended, and our patience with one another, would point to the truth of Jesus and that we actually belong to Him. And sure enough, in God's Word, Jesus turns to His followers and says this about how people will know we belong to Him: "A new commandment I give to you, that you love one another; as I have loved you, that you also love one another. *By this all will know that you are My disciples, if you have love for one another*" (John 13:34–35 NKJV; emphasis added).

> Jesus, the one who made breakfast for His betrayers, wants us to love as He loves.

"Love like Me," He says. "Folks will know you belong to Me because you love each other the same way I've loved you."

Jesus, the one who made breakfast for His betrayers, wants us to love as He loves.

● ● ●

My radio show's producer, Sherri, is African American. She just got back from a trip where she was a guest speaker at a youth event in a church that was primarily white. Just before the Sunday morning service, she was called into the minister's study for prayer, and she met a man who was overtly hostile to her. The way he looked at her, dismissively and contemptuously, made her feel hated. She felt utterly unwelcome, lonely, and out of place.

After she spoke, the same man approached her, took off his glasses, and started crying. He told her that hers was the most influential talk he'd ever heard, and it had affected him particularly because he is very racist against blacks. She was stunned by his honesty.

"We've always been this way. My family has always been racist. I've learned this from my dad. I'm so sorry. I've got to change," he told her. "I can see Jesus is using you. And he's using you to change me."

Sherri then asked to meet his dad. She did. And she hugged him.

I know Sherri takes racism very, very seriously. But, she says, she also has to forgive racists, because she *has* to love people in her family. And they are part of her family. She has to love them as Jesus loves her.

Sherri's love is not naive. But that's exactly why it's so profound. She's setting her offense aside, not because it doesn't matter, not because it isn't completely understandable, but because of what Jesus has done for her. She's choosing against offense, not just because God loves these men but also because God loves her and has set aside her very real offenses in order to be with her.

There are those of us who pat ourselves on the back for loving our families and friends. "I'm loyal to the end; I'd die for my kids," we'll say. Truth is, that's not really terribly remarkable. Everyone, or practically everyone, feels this way.

What *is* terribly remarkable is when someone is willing to love a person, in the name of Jesus, whom he or she would otherwise despise. It makes no sense otherwise. Why would we ever regard someone as family who would otherwise be an enemy? Why ignore his faults, or cover her wrongs with love?

Without Jesus, it simply makes no sense.

Sherri's very refusal, and our very refusal, to take and hold offense is evidence of the existence of God.

This is how they'll know we belong to Him, Jesus says.

So let's love—from this moment forward—because *He* first loved us.

18

ON WINNING—AND BY "WINNING," I MEAN, OF COURSE, LOSING

I've always been Argument Guy.

Argument Guy is the guy everyone hates in college, the one who keeps raising his hand and arguing with the professor. I did it all the way through the University of Illinois. I couldn't help it. I just love logic and philosophy and argument. It keeps me awake.

Everyone else in class was thinking, *Sheesh, dude! Shut up.* And yes, I was aware of that, but I couldn't help myself. I often wanted me to shut up too.

It wasn't just college, either. I got in trouble for arguing with Sunday school teachers, public school teachers, everybody. When I was in fifth grade, I accused Mrs. Throneburg of misleading the students regarding world history. I got kicked out of class in first grade for arguing about the actual "horizon line" with the art lady.

When I was in kindergarten, my mom got a call from my teacher, who had kicked me out of class because I had taken umbrage with her suggestion that Santa Claus existed. I stood up with my professorial eyeglasses and buzz cut and asked her why she was being dishonest with my classmates. I thereby, right then and there, demanded a retraction.

Thankfully, when she called my mom, she was laughing. When a little kid gets all lawyerly, it's cute . . . sort of.

Not so cute at my age now. Oh, I'll argue about anything, and enjoy it. That's my natural disposition, and I'm pretty good at it too. My friends call my style "logical pummeling." I took the LSAT, the law school applications test, and got nearly a perfect score. I heart logic.

Yep, I'm just really good at arguments. I can argue about God, and I almost always win!

And by "win," of course, I mean, "lose."

This is because it just doesn't matter. I hate this, but it's true. Sure, in my fantasy world, I get to out-argue everybody and pin them to the logical mat, and they are so humbled, they turn to me, in tears, and ask what they must do to be saved. They are so in awe of the truth of my premises, validity of my argument, and soundness of my conclusions that they have no choice but to begin their relationship with God.

Yeah, it doesn't work that way. Ever.

Without love, I'm just a bunch of noise. And even when well-intentioned, my arguments are abstractions. People have heard so many words. They want to see the love of God. We quote

Scripture, saying, "God is love," and "Love covers a multitude of sins" (1 John 4:8; 1 Peter 4:8 NLT), but if we don't demonstrate this, our words are just more useless racket.

I'm convinced that this—the battleground of anger and offense, of forgiveness and letting go—is where it all matters. As we noted, this should be no surprise, given what Jesus said should be our defining characteristic: love for one another.

And it's not just love for those who are culturally similar to us. For me, loving someone who's like me is no big deal. Oh, you're a library-loving white guy who's a St. Louis Cardinals fan, and you agree precisely with my anti-elitist politics, and your favorite Muppet is Gonzo, and you also love toast and U2 and ironic humor, and you and your wife memorize lines from *Spinal Tap* together, and you enjoy reading about World War I, and you say you're a Chesterton and C. S. Lewis guy? You're clearly awesome. *I love you.*

But really, so what? Now, try an elitist, annoying activist for a political cause I oppose, with no sense of humor, who prefers Chopra to Chesterton, genuinely thinks Midwesterners are intellectually inferior, and consistently insults people like me. Do I love this person? Not merely tolerate, but actually *love* this person?

If I do, well, we've got something unique and beautiful here. Who says miracles don't still happen?

D. A. Carson says in *Love in Hard Places*:

Ideally, however, the church itself is not made up of natural "friends." It is made up of natural enemies. What binds us together is not common education, common race, common income levels, common politics, common nationality, common accents, common jobs, or anything of the sort.

Christians come together, not because they form a natural collocation, but because they have been saved by Jesus Christ and owe him a common allegiance. In the light of this common allegiance, in light of the fact that they have all been loved by Jesus himself, they commit themselves to doing what he says—and he commands them to love one another. In this light, they are a band of natural enemies who love one another for Jesus' sake.[1]

I hope you caught the part that says, *"in light of the fact that they have all been loved by Jesus himself . . ."*

This is why we can, and should, overlook offenses. This is why we give up our "right" to anger, however justified we feel in it. If I'm to love people the way God loves me, I have to love them faults and all.

It's that simple . . . and that excruciatingly difficult.

● ● ●

Letting go of offense and anger means forgiving, and forgiveness means sacrifice. This is what's so striking to me, as I get older, about Jesus: I'm simultaneously dumbfounded that I'm "off the hook" because of what He's done for me, but still stopped in my tracks by what's being asked of me.

It's both. I know God has already forgiven me. And yet this very truth obligates me. It means if someone has done something to wound me, I have to endure a second hurt, one that feels like another wound. My sense of justice says the person who hurt me should pay; but with forgiveness, it's the forgiver—the victim—who must pay again.

This will probably seem like a silly story, but I'll share it anyway. When I lived in South Florida, I had a surfboard. (This makes little sense, given that I can barely balance myself on dry land, but that's not important now.) My wife loaned it to some friends. They destroyed it, and didn't offer to pay for it.

> Whenever . . . you are willing to forgive, you are saying, "I got this. I'm going to pick up the bill for this."

At that moment, I had a choice: forgive them, and I, and my sense of justice, take the hit, or refuse to forgive them and try to make them pay for it. In either scenario, someone pays.

I'm actually not going to tell you the end of the story, because it doesn't matter. Whenever there's an injury to a relationship, a hurt, a broken heart, or even a broken thing, and you are willing to forgive, you are saying, "I got this. I'm going to pick up the bill for this."

This is, of course, precisely what God has done for us.

Our anger is valuable to us. That's why we want to hold it, to savor it. It means something. It means we've been wronged, we're in the right, and we're the victims in an unfair exchange. We want to even out the scales, and one way to do it, at least psychologically, is to stay offended.

Since anger has value, giving it up requires a sacrifice. And, as we've explored, it's one that's simply not optional for the follower of Jesus. The cross simultaneously stands as a constant reminder of His willingness to "pay the bill," and as an indictment on us when we are unwilling to do the same for others.

● ● ●

There's a story in Luke, where an apparently "good," religious, and rich young man approaches Jesus, wondering what he must do to inherit eternal life. Ultimately, Jesus places a demand on him—sell everything and give to the poor—and we're told the young man heard that and walked away, sad.

I think for many of us who live in this society that is so riven with anger, even addicted to it, Jesus is giving us a similar demand: "Give up your anger. Because of what I've done for you, give it up, and forgive." Sadly, our response is, "That's not fair." And we walk away too.

One thing that strikes me about the rich young man story: Jesus doesn't leave him with room to wriggle. The man will either do what Jesus says, or walk away. There's no splitting the difference, paying lip service, or trying to split theological hairs.

But we love to do this with forgiveness. Jesus tells His followers to forgive as we have been forgiven, yet we find reasons why this doesn't quite apply in our situation. (*Maybe He didn't antici-pate what I was going to have to endure . . . Does He realize what He's asking?*) But we don't walk away sad, like the rich young man.

Instead, we tell ourselves that we can live a Christian life-style, and integrate our own decisions about whom to forgive, and when. This is especially dangerous, because when we do that, we're walking away. But we're not aware we've walked away at all. We've just de-radicalized the very nature of following Jesus, because we think we know a better way.

* * *

So here I am, writing this, knowing full well I'm still struggling with it. I don't come by patience with others easily, or with taking the long view of what God might be doing in their lives. But I'm more patient than I used to be. Yesterday, I inadvertently got in an argument on Twitter. I responded to a well-known actor/comedian who'd tweeted that whenever he talked about his atheism, people told him he shouldn't, because it offends people. I replied that it's too bad, because even though I disagree with him about God, I still love his perspective and his wit.

And that, for some of his followers, was "fightin' words." I have no idea why. But as we went back and forth, I was reminded again of how God is helping me grow up. I didn't need to, or even want to, "win" an exchange. I know there's nothing to win. I knew the people attacking me weren't really attacking *me*. I don't know what they've been through.

We've just de-radicalized the very nature of following Jesus, because we think we know a better way.

I don't have to "win," because I know God is in control, and He loves those people. And I don't have to "win," because there's no status at stake. When people make assertions about me, I can actually think them over, and occasionally say, "You know what? That's a good point."

Of course, there are the direct insults, the verbal slaps. But now, given my understanding of how I should choose to not let them offend me, the whole "turn the other cheek" thing just makes so much sense.

I'm not "winning" or "losing" because I'm not even playing that game anymore. I'm off the board. Jesus is giving us a completely different way to live, and it's one that sets us free from anger, free from ever-present guilt, free to really love people, free from constant anxiety, and free to get a good night's sleep.

19

THE WORLD'S WORST NEIGHBOR

That's me. I'm terrible at neighborhood stuff. I'm aware of this. I don't *like* it, and I'm trying to change it.

Because I'm socially awkward, the last thing I ever want to do is strike up a conversation with the guy walking in the apartment next door. I've got nothing to say. I've even practiced coming up with something. It's really, really hard.

My wife is super-nice by nature. People gravitate to her. I scare people off because I look too intense all the time. I'm a brooder, which sounds cooler than it is. People think I'm deep in thought.

What they suspect I'm thinking about: *What kind of practical validity is there to Kant's categorical imperative?* What I'm actually thinking about: *What kind of bird is Gonzo?*

Anyway, I'm horrible at meeting people, and I don't notice

them very easily, either. I'm kind of oblivious. My Asperger's syndrome has something to do with that, too, but I don't want to use it as an excuse.

So I didn't notice the mom and the stroller. Never. My wife did, but I never noticed her.

One day, the landlord came to our door and told us about the horrible thing that had happened, and my wife tried to describe the young mom to me. "Andrea was the one who took her little baby boy out for a walk all the time, and she was pregnant with her second baby, and her husband's name is Jarrod . . . You don't know who I'm talking about?"

I didn't.

We lived in very tight quarters. All of our units were three stories, but narrow, and we were packed in. I guess I saw lots of people, but I didn't remember anyone because, as I said, I don't talk to people, even if I manage to notice them.

Andrea and Jarrod had been driving back from Andrea's parents' house, her landlord told us. Their little boy was in the backseat. Jarrod swerved to avoid something in the roadway. He drove into a deep ditch, and the car flipped over and sank into the water and Florida muck.

Andrea couldn't get out of the car. Jarrod barely did, through his window. Passing motorists saw the car submerged and flipped it out of the water. The doors were stuck. They couldn't get to Andrea or the boy through the driver's side window. Someone handed Jarrod a shovel. He started hammering away to somehow, someway, get to his pregnant wife and child, trapped in the mud.

The windows were smash-resistant. It took too long.

Andrea died. The little boy had stopped breathing, but CPR saved his life.

"Jarrod's coming back from her funeral today, I guess," their landlord told us. "Just thought you should know, since their unit is directly across the lane."

A couple of days later, Carolyn told me she'd seen Jarrod outside earlier that day, walking with his little boy. She'd not ever spoken with him, but knew from Andrea that he worked out of his own home. So it was just him and his boy in their house, she said, and that must be incredibly lonely.

And I thought about that, and then I did something very un-Brant-like. I got up and walked across the street. I stared at the doorbell, and I waited, and then I pushed it, hoping that no one would answer the door. I didn't know what to say.

I did something very un-Brant-like. I got up and walked across the street.

Jarrod opened the door and stared at me. His little boy was at his legs.

"I'm Brant. I live right there," I said, pointing. "I don't know what to say to you. But my wife and I heard what happened, and we're heartsick for you. I'm so, so sorry."

He just looked at me.

"We're just so sorry," I repeated. "I wanted to tell you that. That's all."

He asked me to come in.

I didn't have to say much, as it turned out. He desperately wanted to just talk about everything. How he and Andrea had met, things she'd enjoyed doing and making, things she'd wanted to do. He showed me pictures. I asked him about her and played with the little boy while he told me about the accident too.

He talked to me for more than two hours.

He asked me if I was religious or something. I told him I was a Christian. He said it makes sense, because his other neighbors run away from him. The ones he'd been social with now just looked at him and looked away and hustled inside their homes.

The next weeks, then months, were excruciating for him. He had wild swings of optimism, despondency, gratitude, and abject rudeness. He wasn't able to be a fun, encouraging friend. It just wasn't possible. He believed in God and was angry at Him. He was crushed with loneliness and loss. He was taxing to be around. And who wouldn't be?

It doesn't matter if I feel stupid. I just want to love people for once.

Amazingly, I kept doing the un-Brant-like thing and kept going back over, kept pushing the doorbell. So not my style.

Jarrod left the neighborhood two years later and moved up north to be near his family and a new romantic interest. It had been exhausting. For two years, Carolyn and I couldn't look out the window without seeing into his first-floor den, where he worked alone, day and night.

We had prayed for him and listened and talked and listened some more.

My wife thought it was an answer to prayer, both that he now had some momentum in his life and that I was getting a break.

Before I'd walked across the street that first time, I thought, *It doesn't even matter what he says to me. And it doesn't matter if I feel stupid. I just want to love people for once.*

When Jarrod asked me if I was religious, I was surprised by

the reaction that, in his mind, it somehow "makes sense" that a Christian would be there. I didn't expect him to say that, and I'm often too quick to criticize our shortcomings as believers. But you know what? It does make sense.

It makes sense that people who follow the Man of Sorrows, a man who was "acquainted with grief," are also acquainted with grief (Isa. 53:3 ESV).

We don't run away from it. We run toward it. And we run toward it knowing full well that people may thrash about, scream, punch, kick, curse, cry, and yell at God and us . . . and then, when they look up, wondering, *Are you still there?* . . . we're still there.

That's because when we're at our best, you can kick and punch, sure, but you can't offend us.

I tell that story with some trepidation because I'm kind of a good guy in my own story. I'm hoping, though, that you realize this spate of others-centeredness is very out of character for me—out of my previous character, anyway. But it made me think, *Maybe I'm growing up. Maybe that's what obedience looks like.*

It may have been something you would do without thinking, like an obvious thing. I don't doubt it. Sometimes it takes me a long time to "get it."

It may also have been obvious to you, for a long time, that "ministry" itself—serving others—*has to involve deciding not to be offended.*

It's not an option. It is the essence of ministry. It finally occurred to me that we can't be agents of healing in people's lives unless we're ready to bear their wounds for them and from them. Looking back, I wonder why it took me so long, how someone who purports to follow Jesus wouldn't have understood this.

He did precisely this for us: bore our wounds, and took a

beating from us, and endured our betrayals. But He was not alienated from us. The disciples who'd abandoned Him looked up, and there He was, on the shore, making breakfast for them.

I want to be like that. When I'm at my best, you can't offend me. When you look up, I want to still be there.

This is ministry itself. I'm not sure there's another kind.

This is what it means to work in a nursing home, among the senile. My grandma was the quintessential bread-baking, flower-growing, sweet-hearted grandma. She served my demanding, rude grandpa for more than a decade, hand and foot, after he endured paralysis and disease. She knew him as a different man. When she looked at him, she saw the man she knew he was and who he could be.

She passed away not long ago, after becoming senile herself. Her nursing home staff was so kind to her. One day, a nurse handed her a glass of orange juice, and my grandma, the sweetest grandma ever, threw it back in her face.

My grandma wasn't herself anymore. A little while later, after Grandma had calmed down, the nurse brought her another juice. That's what servants do. To be in ministry means to choose to be unoffendable.

Ask anyone in ministry to the homeless. Or families who open up homes and hearts to foster children. Or prison ministers. Or people serving troubled kids. Or anyone, anywhere, truly serving anyone.

It's not a side issue, not a secondary concern, not a strategy. Again: *Choosing to be unoffendable out of love for others is ministry.* And real ministry forces us to abandon our relentless search for approval from others.

That frees us to love . . . beautifully and recklessly.

20

IMBALANCED? YOU
BETTER HOPE SO

This story is about me being an idiot. I hope you enjoy it as much as I don't.

Here's what happened:

I bought a new car. First time ever. Still not sure it was a
good idea, but we did it. It gets fifty miles per gallon
because it's a *diesel*, which is unfortunate because . . .
I filled it with regular gas, and that's unfortunate
because . . .
that kinda destroys all the fuel lines and stuff, and that
means . . .
it was going to cost seven grand to fix, which I didn't have,
so . . .

I rode my bike, carrying extra stuff, to work, going uphill
and . . .

managed to injure my back, rendering me bedridden for
several days, and in excruciating pain, so . . .

I'm an idiot.

I felt dumb. And guilty. And stupid. And like a failure. And
some other stuff.

As I rode my bike in difficult weather, I thought, *I deserve
this.* As I lay on the couch, in pain from my bike injury, I thought,
*This is what I get for what I did. I'm paying the price for my screw-
ing this up.* I was doing penance, and I deserved it.

And then Volkswagen called, with the total cost, including
towing, tax, everything: $0.

Nothing. The service guy said the parent company was paying for it. It wasn't a warranty thing. We couldn't make them do it.
They just did it, in hopes of winning long-term customers, I guess.

Zero dollars.

I was happy about this, but here's where it gets weird: *something in me wasn't elated.* There was a part of me—there's *still*
a part of me—that wanted me to pay a price for it. Yes, on one
level, this makes no sense. Maybe you've never felt that way.
Simultaneously thankful and . . . strangely helpless.

I blew it, my wife knew it, and she didn't begrudge it. I blew
it, and the repair guys didn't make me feel stupid. I blew it, and
did something harmful, and didn't pay a dime. What I got, for my
idiocy, was free towing and fixing. And I got a free detailing of the
car, and they changed the oil too. That's what I got.

I had to figure out why this didn't sit entirely well with me: *it
turns out, I hadn't been "paying the price" at all.* I had no control

over this. I'm not being held responsible. Even feeling guilty didn't help. There's nothing about me in this at all.

And that's the problem. It's not about me, not about Brant Hansen.

At. All.

In sports, there's the guy on deck in the bottom of the ninth. He's struck out four times already, but he has—as they say all the time in sports—"a chance to redeem himself" if he gets to the plate. He can still be the hero and win the game for his team.

A chance to "redeem himself."

But I'm the guy who struck out four times, waits on deck for his chance . . . and doesn't get to the plate. The guy in front of me hits the game-winning homer. We win! We're the champions! He did it, not me. I didn't redeem myself. Now I'm sitting in the locker room, and I should be celebrating with everyone else.

● ● ●

Truth is, we find this very, very hard to accept, but *we can't redeem ourselves.* Oh, we like to think we can, deep down, so it's still about us. Carrying around guilt? Still about us. Feeling stupid? Still about us. Feeling like a failure? Still about us. Turning our guilt into seemingly productive energy so we're doing the "right" things? Still about us. Seems so . . . so . . . "righteous," and yet, when we can't take our eyes off ourselves to celebrate the win, it's just plain about us. That's pride.

And pride always hurts, but it's positively deadly when masked by our attempts to pay our own way with our religious activity.

The game is over. We're still on the religious playing field, still trying to redeem ourselves.

And God is popping the cork.

●　●　●

Choosing to be an unoffendable person is not "common sense." It is not normal to practice a lifestyle of letting go of one's "right" to anger—even at oneself. The whole thing sounds unfair, imbalanced, and out of step with how the world usually operates.

And so does grace. It's completely unfair. It's imbalanced in the highest degree. And—thank God—it's utterly out of step with how the world usually operates.

This is why grace itself offends the self-righteous. Remarkably, I found it hard to take, even when grace was shown to *me*, by the VW folks. I so wanted to be my own redeemer. This is the normal way of things. This is how the world works.

And how the world "works" is often what we perceive to be the "balanced" position, the one that leaves the status quo intact. As I've listened to objections to the subject of this book, I've heard much about "balance," such as, "Sure, we need to forgive, but we need to balance that with knowing when it's often healthy to stay angry," and so forth.

Let's stay "balanced." Of course. Yes.

Now, please know, I'm not Mr. Extreme by nature. I'm Mr. So-Not-Extreme, actually. Happy to meet you. I'd love to be that guy who writes those awesome books about being incredibly cool and jumping off cliffs on a mountain bike or running with the bulls while on fire or whatever. I admire that rock-climber guy who got trapped and cut off his own arm. That guy's extreme. I don't even have any tats. That's how lame I am.

I have a mountain bike . . . with a basket on the front. That way I can carry my bag of peas to work each day in the basket. I'm not kidding about this. I repeat: *I carry a bag of peas to work each day in my bike basket.*

I'm not a big risk-taker. I don't care for spicy food. I eat stacks of toast, with nothing on it. Just stacks of plain toast. Put a picture of that on a motivational poster. That car I was talking about earlier? It's a station wagon. My brother lettered in practically every high school sport; I lettered in—again, not kidding, I seriously got letters for this—keeping statistics. When they took a team picture, I was the guy in street clothes, kneeling with a clipboard.

You love the *Fast and Furious* films? I seriously watch documentaries about sloths.

Anyway, the point is this: I *like* being reasonable. I *like* telling people not to get too crazy with their ideas. I *like* reeling people back in. I *like* balance! But there's a problem: None of this "balance" talk is scriptural language. None. Because the way the world works and the kingdom that Jesus describes are squarely at odds.

> I *like* balance! But there's a problem: None of this "balance" talk is scriptural language.

The kingdom of God knows nothing of "balance." It's as balanced as, say, a teeter-totter with a gnat on one side and a hippo with, say, a grand piano on the other. No, wait; that's misleading. The gnat has to move. It's a teeter-totter with *nothing* on one end, and a hippo, grand piano, and also a gnat, because I just moved the gnat over there.

In the economy of the kingdom of God, we can't even afford the gnat. The kingdom is not "balanced," it doesn't operate via our "common sense," and you can't possibly, try as you might, "take it too far."

Being a citizen of that kingdom, then, means operating in that whole new economy, and grace—unfair, imbalanced grace—is the currency.

By the way, I've learned it's worth reminding that extending grace does not mean, and has never meant, that there is "no such thing as sin," or that there's no such thing as right or wrong, or that God smiles on all of our actions. There is sin, there is right and wrong, and God, like any loving father, of course cares about what we do and who we are.

But that's why grace is "grace." It amazes us because we really *don't* deserve it, because we really *have* failed, because there really *is* so much reason for God to walk away from us, instead of running toward us.

God doesn't love all the things we do. He loves us in spite of the things we do.

So let's do something crazy and imbalanced here: let's embrace the unfairness.

Why? Because not only is it in our best interest, but also, frankly, *Jesus gives us no other option.*

In Matthew, Jesus tells a story about a business that hires workers, and it's a wonderful business. It's so wonderful that it makes people just plain mad:

> "The kingdom of heaven is like a person who owned some land. One morning, he went out very early to hire some people to work in his vineyard. The man agreed to pay the

workers one coin for working that day. Then he sent them into the vineyard to work. About nine o'clock the man went to the marketplace and saw some other people standing there, doing nothing. So he said to them, 'If you go and work in my vineyard, I will pay you what your work is worth.' So they went to work in the vineyard. The man went out again about twelve o'clock and three o'clock and did the same thing. About five o'clock the man went to the marketplace again and saw others standing there. He asked them, 'Why did you stand here all day doing nothing?' They answered, 'No one gave us a job.' The man said to them, 'Then you can go and work in my vineyard.'

"At the end of the day, the owner of the vineyard said to the boss of all the workers, 'Call the workers and pay them. Start with the last people I hired and end with those I hired first.'

"When the workers who were hired at five o'clock came to get their pay, each received one coin. When the workers who were hired first came to get their pay, they thought they would be paid more than the others. But each one of them also received one coin. When they got their coin, they complained to the man who owned the land. They said, 'Those people were hired last and worked only one hour. But you paid them the same as you paid us who worked hard all day in the hot sun.' But the man who owned the vineyard said to one of those workers, 'Friend, I am being fair to you. You agreed to work for one coin. So take your pay and go. I want to give the man who was hired last the same pay that I gave you. I can do what I want with my own money. Are you jealous because I am good to those people?'

"So those who are last now will someday be first, and those who are first now will someday be last." (20:1–16 NCV)

"Do you begrudge my generosity?" the landowner is saying.

The answer, of course, is yes, they do. They begrudge it quite a bit. Even though it has no impact on them whatsoever, it offends them. We hate it when we are trying so hard to earn something, and then someone else gets the same thing without trying as hard.

Think about this for a moment, in real, "today" terms. Someone gives you a backbreaking job, and you're happy for it, but at the end of the day, when you're getting paid, the guys who came in with five minutes left get the same amount you just got. Seriously?

It's imbalanced, unfair, maddening . . . *and it's also exactly what Jesus just said the kingdom of God is like.*

Not only is it maddening; it's maddening to the "good" people! Common sense says you don't do this. You don't pay latecomers who came in a few minutes ago the same amount that you paid the hardworking folks you hired first. Jesus tells this story, knowing full well that the conscientious ones listening would find this hardest to take.

And, as a matter of fact, as a conscientious one, I find this hard to take. I'm just being honest. This story does not fit my style. I'm all about people getting what they deserve.

Oh, it's offensive, too, when Jesus turns to a guy who's being executed next to Him, and tells him, "Today, you will be with me in paradise" (Luke 23:43). What did the guy do to deserve that? He did nothing.

If you call yourself a Christian, and you want things to be

fair, and you want God's rewards given out only to the deserving and the upstanding and the religious, well, honestly, Jesus has got to be a complete embarrassment to you.

In fact, to so many upstanding Christians, He is. He has always been offensive, and remains offensive, to those who seek to achieve "righteousness" through what they do. Always.

People who've grown up in church (like me) are well acquainted with the idea that Jesus is our "cornerstone." He's the solid rock of our faith. Got it. Not controversial. It's well-known. But what's not so talked about: That stone, Jesus, causes religious people to stumble. And that rock is offensive to "good" people:

> So what does all this mean? Those who are not Jews were not trying to make themselves right with God, but they were made right with God because of their faith. The people of Israel tried to follow a law to make themselves right with God. But they did not succeed, because they tried to make themselves right by the things they did instead of trusting in God to make them right. They stumbled over the stone that causes people to stumble. (Rom. 9:30–32 NCV)

And then Paul says something a couple verses later that angers "good Christians" to this day:

> Because they did not know the way that God makes people right with him, they tried to make themselves right in their own way. So they did not accept God's way of making people right. Christ ended the law so that everyone who believes in him may be right with God. (Rom. 10:3–4 NCV)

It's not subtle, what Paul's writing here. For anyone who believes in Him, Jesus *ended the law* as a means to righteousness.

Yet so many think they can achieve—even have achieved— some kind of "good Christian" status on the basis of the rule-keeping work they've done. They suspect they'll do good things and God will owe them for it, like payment for a job well done. Paul says, in effect, if you think you should get what you earn, you will . . . and you don't want that.

> When people work, their pay is not given as a gift, but as something earned. But people cannot do any work that will make them right with God. So they must trust in him, who makes even evil people right in his sight. Then God accepts their faith, and that makes them right with him. (Rom. 4:4–5 NCV)

Think about this: This is extremely offensive to anyone with typical religious sensibilities. In this scripture, the one who does not work is in better shape with God than the worker, if that one simply believes in the God who justifies ungodly people.

This is why I put "good Christians" in quotes: there are none.

This is why I put "good Christians" in quotes: there are none.

Yes, upstanding, moral people trip over this rock. People are trying so hard, and hoping so much, that by being good they can be considered righteous before God. Everything about Jesus says to abandon this project, humble yourself, and believe in the God who "justifies the ungodly" (Rom. 4:5).

This is not how religions are supposed to work. Heck, it's not how *anything* is supposed to work. As we talked about in an earlier chapter, even irreligious people come up with their own rules for being "good" and judge others according to those rules. It's how we operate, how the world works.

You're supposed to get what's coming to you based on how you keep the rules. It's the common-sense thing. It's, you know, "balanced."

Jesus is imbalanced.

You'd better be glad.

21

I CAN WORSHIP A GOD LIKE THAT

Once upon a time, there was a prostitute. She lived in Hawaii, and it was her birthday. Her name was Agnes. Tony Campolo writes about her in his book *The Kingdom of God Is a Party.*

He was in a diner in Honolulu, very late one night—three thirty in the morning, actually—when he couldn't sleep from jet lag. It was just him, his donut and coffee, and the guy behind the counter, when suddenly, a group of prostitutes came in. They sat down on either side of Tony, and they were very crude and very loud. He was about to leave.

But then he overheard one of them saying tomorrow was her birthday, her thirty-ninth. Another woman made fun of her for bringing it up. "What do you want, Agnes, a party? You want a cake? You want us to sing 'Happy Birthday'?"

Agnes said no, she didn't. She'd never had a party, or a birthday cake, so why start now?

When I heard that, I made a decision. I sat and waited until the women had left. Then I called over the fat guy behind the counter, and I asked him, "Do they come in here every night?"

"Yeah!" he answered.

"The one right next to me, does she come here every night?"

"Yeah!" he said. "That's Agnes. Yeah, she comes in here every night. Why d'ya wanta know?"

"Because I heard her say that tomorrow is her birthday," I told him. "What do you say you and I do something about that? What do you think about us throwing a birthday party for her—right here—tomorrow night?"[1]

The guy behind the counter—his name was Harry—loved the idea, and so did his wife, who did the cooking in back. In fact, he wanted to make the birthday cake.

Tony told him he'd be there earlier the next morning, in time to decorate. And he decorated, complete with crepe paper streamers and a sign that read, "Happy Birthday, Agnes!"

Apparently, word of the party got out, because the place was filled with prostitutes before Agnes's arrival. When she came in at three-thirty with a friend, the whole place erupted, "Happy birthday!"

She was stunned. Mouth agape. "Flabbergasted," Tony writes. Her friend had to steady her. And when they began to sing, she began to cry.

Harry lit the candles, and as she blew out the cake, she was in tears. She didn't want to cut it. Instead, she asked if she could keep it a little while. She wondered if that would be okay.

Harry said she could. Then she said, "I want to take the cake home, okay? I'll be right back, honest!"

She left. Everyone was stunned silent. Tony said he didn't know what else to do, so he broke the silence with, "What do you say we pray?"

> Looking back on it now, it seems more than strange for a sociologist to be leading a prayer meeting with a bunch of prostitutes in a diner in Honolulu at 3:30 in the morning. But then it just felt like the right thing to do.
>
> I prayed for Agnes. I prayed for her salvation. I prayed that her life would be changed and that God would be good to her.
>
> When I finished, Harry leaned over the counter and with a trace of hostility in his voice, he said, "Hey! You never told me you were a preacher. What kind of church do you belong to?"
>
> In one of those moments when just the right words came, I answered, "I belong to a church that throws birthday parties for whores at 3:30 in the morning."
>
> Harry waited a moment and then almost sneered as he answered, "No you don't. There's no church like that. If there was, I'd join it. I'd join a church like that!"[2]

You know what? I have a new rule: I won't join a church that *doesn't* do that. Because that's the Jesus I recognize, the One who mends the brokenhearted and is never, ever scandalized by sinners.

The Founder of my faith gave us new rules of engagement. He was told, like everyone else in His society, to stay away from lepers. He wouldn't do it. Sure, it made people mad that Jesus was flouting their rules. But He didn't stay away from lepers. Instead, He touched them and made them whole.

Crowds grumbled at Him when they saw His choice of company, like a man who worked with the occupying Roman government to steal their money from them. They watched Jesus even invite Himself over to Zacchaeus's house—a nice house that, no doubt, was purchased using their own stolen money.

Of course they grumbled. He had dinner, too—on their dime, they realized—and it sent all the wrong messages. Surely there were children in the crowd, too, who might "have gotten the wrong idea"—you know, that we should hang around people like that. (People upset about grace always trot that one out: "Sure, *I* understand, but kids could get the impression it's okay to eat dinner with tax thieves, and so you really shouldn't do that." Sure. They're always concerned about "the kids.")

I wonder if the crowd heard Him call out to Zacchaeus, and if they thought, *Oh, yeah, this is going to be good. He's going to let him have it!*—and then they heard Jesus honor him by inviting Himself over for dinner. No wonder they grumbled. I bet they flat-out booed.

And as it turns out . . . Zacchaeus's heart was changed. It didn't take a big, blasting speech from Jesus at the dinner table, either. The very fact that Jesus *wasn't offended* by him, and would be with him, and would show love to him in front of others, and would sit in his dining room—*that* changed his heart.

And that's just it: it's always grace that changes hearts.

Rules are wonderful. As I said in chapter 2, I'm a rules guy.

Rules bring wisdom into our lives. They help us live better. They spare us from pain.

But rules don't change anyone's heart, ever.

Grace does.

To paraphrase Harry, the diner guy in Tony Campolo's story: "Wait—a God who picks the guy with the worst reputation, doesn't care, and invites Himself over for dinner in front of a self-righteous crowd? I could worship a God like that."

Rules don't change anyone's heart, ever. Grace does.

* * *

A guy once asked me to go with him to Indonesia to help people after the latest tsunami hit. I said yes. I had no idea what I was doing.

We arrived in Banda Aceh two weeks after the destruction. (Indonesia alone lost a mind-bending two hundred thousand lives.)

We weren't welcomed by everyone. Most people love the help, sure. But I felt unwelcome when a group of Muslim separatists threatened to kill us. (I have a sixth sense about this kind of thing.)

They were opposed to Western interference in Aceh and didn't want us saying anything about Jesus. I just wanted to help some people. I also wanted a hotel. I wanted a safer place. I didn't want to die. I had no idea what I was getting into.

We took supplies to what was, before the tsunami, a fishing village. It was now a group of people living on the ground, some in tents.

I just followed what the rest of our little group was doing. They had more experience. We distributed the food, housewares, cooking oil, that sort of thing, and stayed on the ground with them. That's how our little disaster-response group operated, even though I wanted a hotel. They stayed among the victims and lived with them.

After the militant group threatened to slit our throats, I felt kind of vulnerable out there, lying on the ground. As a dad with two little kids, I didn't sign up for the martyr thing. I took the threat seriously and wanted to leave.

The local imam resisted our presence, too, and this bugged me. "Well, if you hate us, maybe we should leave. It's a thousand degrees, we've got no AC or running water or electricity, and your co-religionists are threatening us. So, yeah. Maybe let's call it off." But it wasn't up to me, and I didn't have a flight back.

As we helped distribute supplies to nearby villages, people repeatedly asked the same question: "Why are you here?" They simply couldn't understand *why* we would be there with them. They told us they thought we were enemies.

One of the members of our group spent time working in a truck with locals, driving slowly through the devastation, in the sticky humidity, picking up the bodies of their neighbors. They piled them in the back of a truck.

It was horrific work. They wore masks, of course, but there's no covering the smell of death.

The locals paused and asked him too: "Why? Why are you here?"

He told them it was because he worshiped Jesus, and he was convinced that Jesus would be right there, in the back of the truck with them. He loves them.

"But you are our enemy."

"Jesus told us to love our enemies."

The imam eventually warmed up to us, and before we left, he even invited our little group to his home for dinner! We sat in his home, one of the few in the area still standing. He explained through an interpreter that he didn't trust us at first, because we were Christians. But while other "aid" groups would drive by, throw a box out of a car, and get their pictures taken with the people of his village, our group was different.

We slept on the ground.

He knew we'd been threatened, he knew we weren't comfortable, and he knew we didn't have to be there. But there we were, his supposed enemies, and we would not be offended. We would not be alienated. We were on the ground with his people.

His wives peered in from the kitchen, in tears. He passed around a trophy with the photo of a twelve-year-old boy, one of his children. He told us the boy had been lost in the tsunami, and could we please continue to search for him? Was there anything we could do? We were crying too.

We looked at the trophy, given to the boy for his excellent Koran memorization skills.

The imam then said something that shocked us all, and even in the intervening years, still boggles my mind: He asked us to take his remaining kids—they were sitting in the room with us—and raise them as our own in America. He knew they would be better off, he said.

He offered us . . . his children? We looked at each other. *Did we just hear that right?*

We did. And we didn't know how to react. We were heart-broken by the desperation. We knew the legalities made the idea immediately impossible. I don't remember how that conversation ended. I know we left, and it hurt to leave.

I remember all of us talking afterward about a lot of things, like how dangerous it might be for him to even make that offer. Or how desperate they must be to survive right now. The most puzzling thing: How is it even possible that someone could go from "You're my sworn enemy; you're not welcome here," to "I want you to raise my children"?

As I said, I'm still stunned. How does a heart change like that? The only thing I can think is he saw love. He knew we loved his people. I don't know what else does that.

We can love; we can forgive; we can refuse to be offended . . . because God loved us first. Even in our weakness, even overlooking the disaster scene that is humanity, He was not alienated. He proved it. He took on our flesh and dwelt among us. He embraced our brokenness, our smell, even our death.

He got in the back of the truck with us.

The imam and the villagers didn't have a heart change because of logical argument, or anything except, I think, that they got a glimpse of Jesus.

The Jesus they saw loves people. Without regard, He loves them. And when nightmares sweep people's lives away, leaving them helpless, on the ground, He lies down next to them.

●　●　●

I went to an aquarium once at a major metropolitan zoo that had all sorts of helpful signs. They all had a similar theme: *all animal species, everywhere, are in jeopardy, and it's mankind's fault.* I just wanted to see stripey fish that glowed and stuff.

Anyway, I stopped in front of one display and reread the sign. Did it really just say that?

Yep, it said: "The fish in this display are all native to the South Pacific Ocean. We have removed the predators, so you can observe the fish relating in peace as they do in nature."

Okay. Think about that.

Yeah, I guess if you take out all predators, all the fish live in peace, just like in the ocean . . . where there are predators.

Nope. Makes no sense whatsoever. It's boring too. And certainly not "natural."

The world isn't safe like that. We can play pretend and try to set up an aquarium-type existence, devoid

We can play pretend and try to set up an aquarium-type existence, devoid of interaction with anything or anyone who might challenge or upset us, but that's not the world Jesus came to save.

of interaction with anything or anyone who might challenge or upset us, but that's not the world Jesus came to save. He entered the violent one, the brutal one.

●　●　●

I really do feel that God is helping me grow up. The things Jesus said make more sense to me now, and I understand better what Paul wrote about getting rid of all anger. The point isn't that we were justified in our anger. The point is freedom—freedom to love. Freedom to have God-given sight, the ability to look at that highly offensive someone and see what is not yet, as though it were.

We're made for it, so we'll find it both exhausting . . . and exhilarating.

Henri Nouwen was a priest. He also had plenty of what the culture considers "significant": he was a brilliant writer and a professor at both Yale and Harvard. As he lived his life, he saw the struggle between operating by the values of the world and the values of the kingdom of God.

> More and more, the desire grows in me simply to walk around, greet people, enter their homes, sit on their doorsteps, play ball, throw water, and be known as someone who wants to live with them. It is a privilege to have the time to practice this simple ministry of presence.
>
> Still, it is not as simple as it seems. My own desire to be useful, to do something significant, or to be part of some impressive project is so strong that soon my time is taken up by meetings, conferences, study groups, and workshops that prevent me from walking the streets. It is difficult not to have plans, not to organize people around an urgent cause, and not to feel that you are working directly for social progress.
>
> But I wonder more and more if the first thing shouldn't be to know people by name, to eat and drink with them, to listen to their stories and tell your own, and to let them know with words, handshakes, and hugs that you do not simply like them, but truly love them.[3]

Loving people means divesting ourselves of our status. We're not being naive in doing it. We've surrendered it for good reason, believing that there is something better in exchange. We decide to be unoffendable because that's how love operates; it gives up its "status" entirely.

I'm not overstating this. In the book of Philippians, Paul tells us to consider others more significant than ourselves. We are to have the same mind as Jesus: "He did not think that being equal with God was something to be used for his own benefit. But he gave up his place with God and made himself nothing. He was born as a man and became like a servant" (2:6–7 NCV).

God showed us how to love. And He did it, even though He is a king, choosing not to be born in a palace. Imagine the headline: "King of Kings Born, Immediately Placed in Feeding Trough."

That's the Jesus of the Back of the Truck.

And yes, I can worship a God like that.

HERE'S THE PART WHERE I TALK ABOUT SOME DANISH PEOPLE

There's this great movie, made from a book, called *Babette's Feast*, and it's set in a Danish fishing village.[1] At least I think that's where it's set. It's really foggy, and I can't understand Danish. I first read about it in Philip Yancey's life-changing book *What's So Amazing About Grace?* and decided to give it a try.[2]

It's about these two beautiful young ladies and their joyless father, who is pastor of his own religious group. They live a spartan, severe life, devoid of pleasures, in accordance with his teachings. They have opportunities to marry good men, but their father sends the young men packing. The sisters wind up elderly single ladies, still devoted to their father's religion, and now leading a dying little group of uptight, aging, true believers.

One rainy night, a young woman comes to their door, begging for help, and they let her in. She's a refugee from war-torn Paris, and she becomes their maid and cook, and serves them for years . . . until she wins the lottery.

She takes all of her lottery winnings and uses them for one purpose: making the most ridiculously fabulous meal imaginable for the old ladies and their congregation. Unbeknownst to the sisters, she happens to be one of the greatest chefs in the world, who had made her name at a restaurant in France before she was forced to leave.

Shipments arrive in the little village from all over the world, each with an exotic ingredient for the great meal. She prepares buckwheat cakes with caviar, turtle soup, her signature *Caille en Sarcophage avec Sauce Perigourdine*—quail in pastry with foie gras and truffle sauce—and an endless list of other specialties. (By the way, I looked this stuff up. I'd have no idea what this is otherwise.)

Of course, she also serves the most rare and delicious wines and champagnes. She serves the entire meal on the fine china she'd ordered, with new linens and crystal.

Her entire lottery winnings, gone—for one meal. For one magnificent, mind-blowing blessing.

The ladies see what's happening, of course, as she prepares all this, and they don't like it. They're not comfortable with all this preparation for deliciousness and enjoyment. It's just not right, you know.

They decide, along with their little congregation, for whom Babette is preparing the tastiest meal of a lifetime, to eat it but not enjoy it. They realize it's a gift, but they don't have to like it. It wouldn't be right.

They sit. They eat, slowly and suspiciously at first. They eye one another, making sure no one is enjoying this too much. But it's too good. It's all just too good. The setting, the atmosphere, the soup, the wine . . . it's spectacular. Joy breaks out.

There's another guest at the meal, a former suitor of one of the sisters, who's now a general. And he knows Paris, knows great meals, and recognizes this one for what it is—the work of a master. He knows the chef must surely be the one and only Babette, formerly of the world-renowned Café Anglais.

He realizes, too, that this sumptuous meal, prepared for people previously unwilling to embrace it, is, purely and simply, grace.

"Mercy imposes no conditions. And, lo! Everything we have chosen has been granted to us, and everything we rejected has also been granted. Yes, we even get back what we rejected. For mercy and truth are met together, and righteousness and bliss shall kiss one another," he proclaims.[3]

It's such a brilliant story, and I hope you watch the movie, even if you're not big on the whole foggy-Danish-fishing-village genre of film. You'll likely find yourself wondering, *What's wrong with these people? Just relax and enjoy the great gifts you've been given!*

And maybe you'll recognize yourself in them.

● ● ●

It takes a childlike humility to embrace the love of God, to realize how "unfair" it is, and then add, quickly, "but I'll take it!"

Especially after a lifetime of carefully measuring everyone's actions, comparing ourselves to them, observing people to make sure they're not getting away with anything, and just generally trying to control and evaluate everything, well . . .

> **It takes a childlike humility to embrace the love of God, to realize how "unfair" it is, and then add, quickly, "but I'll take it!"**

it's quite a switch. And it can sure be offensive. *I worked so hard and they get paid the same as me? The guy on the cross gets to steal from people and party or who-knows-what and suddenly he's going to paradise?*

We can resent it, trip over it, or try to explain away the scandal of it, in hopes of making Jesus fit into our more equitable ideals. But if we do this, instead of humbling ourselves and just thanking God for how wonderful He is to us, we're setting ourselves up for a lifetime of offense, because we'll never, ever feel secure with God.

God wants us to accept gifts. It takes humility to do it, which is why kids are so much better than we are at this. No kid balks at a gift. No eight-year-old opens a PlayStation on Christmas morning and says, "No—I just can't. I don't deserve this. I am unworthy. No. Take it back."

It takes humility, and accepting the world-saving unfairness of the kingdom is no different. Accept it. Breathe it in. You might finally be able to relax, not have to worry about how you "measure up," and then you can actually focus on other people.

Or you can try to explain the scandal of grace away, make it more "reasonable" and "balanced," and refuse to enjoy the finest meal ever prepared.

● ● ●

Living in humility is refreshing. It's also incredibly difficult, at times, because it means trusting—*really* trusting. And that's hard to do. Read what one listener had to say:

Brant,

I listen to your show and have noticed that you tackle a lot of issues and thoughts that most people avoid when discussing Christianity. I appreciate your honesty and thought-provoking commentary on Jesus. In saying that I thought you might have a thought on something that I am struggling with:

In the Bible Jesus says, "My yoke is easy and my burden is light" (Matthew 11:30). I feel like my walk with God can be really difficult at times. I know Jesus paid for my sins but I constantly feel guilty about bad decisions I have made in the past as well as the daily struggles I face as a human. I guess in a way I don't understand how God can constantly extend His grace to someone who messes up so much.

Thoughts?

Jacob

Hey Jacob!

Great question. I've certainly felt this way before. I think most have.

An odd thing I noticed: When *The Passion of the Christ*, the movie, came out, I remember so many people saying, "Why'd Jesus have to put up with *all* of that? Why was it so bad? Why did He have to be flogged, and mocked, and spat upon, and beat up, and nailed up in front of everyone, and then speared, and . . ."

And then, later, when we're considering our sinfulness, we find ourselves asking, "Can God *really* forgive me? I've done so much wrong, and over and over, and . . ."

We should connect those two things. When we consider our sinfulness, consider what God has done for us. Is there anything left, anything He didn't cover? Are we so bad that Jesus needs to suffer again? Did He not go far enough to cover *my* rebellion? Or yours?

No way. I'm not that special, and neither are you. There's not one thing left undone, not one more punishment God has to take on our behalf, to meet the demands of the Law. Nothing.

"It is finished," Jesus said. The Law has been fulfilled, completed. Done. And if that was too subtle, the curtain that divided God from the sinners was ripped in two.

And this is why, too, Jesus said those needing rest could come to Him and find it. People are positively beaten down with guilt, beaten down with the demands of religions, including the Christian one, and feeling like they can *never* measure up. This is because they can't. But Jesus can.

He fulfilled the Law on our behalf. The work is done now, and it's not about what Jacob does, or Brant does, but about *what Jesus already DID*. Price paid, and in full. There's nothing left. Some people won't like this. They're afraid if you believe this, if everyone believes this, everything will turn to chaos. They think once you realize how good God really is, you'll be out of control.

They'll say, "Now grace is great, but . . ." Grace, *but* . . .

Beware of those people.

There is no "but." If you've put on Christ, there is no. more. condemnation. And as we grow in love for God, as we realize we are no longer under law but led by the Spirit, good stuff flows from us!

His "yoke" is easy, and the burden is light, for those who understand this. It does not mean that living a life of love will always be easy—forgiving others never is. It does mean that Jesus' "yoke," His teachings, are not the complex, here's-how-you-keep-the-law-better teachings that so many rabbis offered. Love the Lord your God with all you have, and love your neighbor. That sums it all up. That's how He wants us to live.

And your "righteousness" isn't the issue. *His is*. Final answer. Weirdly, this is also a blow to those of us who grew up suspecting that we weren't pleasing God *unless* we felt kinda guilty. We want it to be about us. But it's not.

Use your guilt to drive you back to Jesus, to drive you back to this truth, that for those in Christ, there is no condemnation. Use your guilt for that . . . and then drop it.

The pressure's off. Soak it in. Take a deep breath. You know what? Letting go of all that guilt because of the gospel, the "news that brings joy," can free you up to be even more of a blessing to people.

And you will be!

Best,

Brant

It's no wonder we're so uptight, so unwilling to be graceful toward people, so quick to be offended, and so lightning-fast to justify our offense as "righteous anger." If we're insecure in our own position with God, there's no way we can begin to relax, not even for a moment. We simply must be vigilant.

So we have a choice: be offended by Jesus Himself, or embrace the breathtaking unfairness of the kingdom. The unfairness of it all is exactly what the older, jealous brother was complaining about in Jesus' story about the prodigal son. There's something in us that wants our salvation to come through us. We don't like being on the sidelines while someone else wins the game.

Again, it's not like any of this is new. The scripture Paul referred to—"Behold, I am laying in Zion a stone of stumbling, and a rock of offense" (Rom. 9:33 ESV)—dates back to centuries before Christ. It's in the book of Isaiah (see 8:14; 28:16).

Many of us would rather go down on our own terms than be humble. It's that simple, and it's that tragic.

We humans can't save ourselves, but we want to be our own saviors. And many of us would rather go down on our own terms than be humble. It's that simple, and it's that tragic.

Jesus has been offensive for centuries. Blessed, indeed, are those who aren't offended by Him. They're the ones who can become like little kids and just know a great gift when they see it. They don't have to pose.

They can simply accept an invitation to the greatest feast of all, and they can enjoy every minute of it.

23

FORGET DANISH PEOPLE—LET'S TALK ABOUT YOUR ELBOW

I want to talk about your elbow precisely because you're not thinking about it right now. That is, at least until I mentioned it you weren't thinking about your elbow, unless you just injured it, or it's bruised or inflamed or something. If there's something wrong with it, sure, it's on your mind. That's the point.

I have some kind of shoulder issue at the moment, and if I move it much at all, or something touches it, it hurts. (Yes, I should go to the doctor for this, but [a] I'm a guy, and [b] I'd rather just search online and come up with the worst possible medical scenarios and freak myself out. This is my plan.) Because of the inflammation, I'm acutely aware of my right shoulder. I'm always thinking about it, adjusting for it, even changing my plans to avoid hurting it.

Timothy Keller uses the idea of favoring an inflamed joint to make a great point: this is precisely how the human ego works. It "hurts" when it's inflamed. Sure, it's always there—everyone's got an ego—but when it's oversized, it's constantly being injured or threatened. When it's "all about me," I'm constantly aware of myself, bracing myself for ego injury.[1]

Real humility isn't about putting yourself down or pretending your performance is substandard at everything you try. Real humility lies in self-forgetfulness.

Few want to hear this, but it's true, and it can be enormously helpful in life: if you're constantly being hurt, offended, or angered, you should honestly evaluate your inflamed ego.

When you're humble, you're not constantly thinking, *How do I look?* or *Am I a success?* or *What do they think of me?* It's just not on your radar screen. When self-interested thoughts do cross your mind, you're able to recognize them for what they are, in most cases: downright silly.

If you're constantly being hurt, offended, or angered, you should honestly evaluate your inflamed ego.

I noticed something about my grandma when she was in her eighties. She was very sweet and intelligent, and even had a job in addition to doing all the typical grandma stuff. She seemed younger than her years. But what I noticed was that, simply put, when it came to people's opinions of her, Grandma just didn't care.

It wasn't rudeness, and she was still servant-hearted. So far as I could tell, she was just completely unconcerned with whether people thought she was "successful" in life. She'd always been brilliant with flowers, and she still planted them everywhere, but no one who knew her thought it was to impress anyone. She delighted in growing things.

I wrote this when she turned ninety:

My grandma don't care what you think.

No offense, she just doesn't. Nothing personal. Wreatha Peters turned ninety last week, and you may have noticed, ninety-year-olds don't really give a rip about their approval ratings. Ninety-year-olds aren't fashionable, and it's not because they can't get to the mall. They just plain don't care. And—let's face it—when you don't care what other people think, you don't tend to go to the mall.

A well-established concept in psychology is the "imaginary audience," and one particularly great experiment plumbing this had college students, given new T-shirts, attending a large lecture. The shirts had oversized, and embarrassing, pictures of Barry Manilow's face. After the class, they were asked, "What percentage of fellow students noticed you?" They all guessed around 80 percent.

Reality: almost no one noticed.[2]

To be young is to be attuned to the adoring, or mocking, crowd that isn't. To be attuned, and to care, deeply. But Grandma? No caring. Grandma's imaginary audience done got up and went.

Her hearing is fine, but applause is a waste of time, honestly. You'll just sting your hands. Applause only means something to us when we're young, because applause, at its deepest level, *bodes something* for us: some future advance in station, some future payoff, some future . . . something . . . that will make us more powerful, more able to get what we want, and maybe(!) that something will satisfy us.

Applause is a promissory note.

When you're old and wiser, you don't accept promissory notes. You're too smart. You know you're going to die, and it's not going to matter. Earlier in life, you knew that, too, but you didn't allow yourself to think about it.

Poet Austin Dobson once wrote, "Fame is a food that dead men eat."

Grandma isn't hungry anymore.[3]

● ● ●

Once, a friend invited me to a fancy conference in Washington, DC. I really had no business there. But I found myself in this hotel suite, where they were having a reception for some leaders from African governments. The suite had one of those lunch meat 'n' crackers–type spreads out. Since I have poor social skills and like crackers, I spent a lot of time in the lunch meat 'n' crackers area.

Anyway, I overheard this lady, who was going from government leader guy to government leader guy, explaining what God had told her to do, which was to save the world. That was her mandate, and she told them she was going to start small: with Africa. She had a Big Vision, and she was going to do this and that, and then this other thing, and then this would happen, and she had it pretty much mapped out. It was awesome.

I like people who can rescue everybody, so I thought to myself, *That's cool*, and then I noticed they had those fancy

Pepperidge Farm cookie-stix things. I also noticed she moved on to the next guy and talked a lot again about what she was going to do. She had some big plans that involved her doing some significant stuff. Pretty neat.

It was lunchtime, so I made my way to this big lunch area downstairs, where they had more crackers. The lunch organizers had arranged for a young married couple to speak. The guy never spoke, actually. His wife said he was more of the computer-nerd type, and she was nervous, but she'd talk, since they asked.

She is a Jesus-follower who had gone to Africa (Africa, again?) awhile back for a few weeks. She made some friends there who didn't have much of anything. When she came back, she asked God to help her help them. And she got an idea: she and her husband scanned their wedding guest list into their computer and asked those folks to loan their African friends some money. Her husband set up a website so their wedding friends could loan the money and make contact with the people they were giving to.

She didn't know what else to do. This couple was heartbroken for a few families, and she knew God loved them. They had no Big Vision, just love for a few people she knew, and she wanted to help them start businesses so they could have some way to live.

God blessed their efforts.

They've now helped more than a few people. They've helped hundreds of thousands. More than a million people have loaned money through them, and it's added up to more than five hundred *million* dollars.

She said they didn't really know what they were doing—they just loved a few people. She doesn't understand how this happened, she said, except she thinks God made it happen.

I didn't walk away from that lunch impressed at how amazingly talented the couple was. Instead, I thought about how God loves us, and how He favors the underdog.

He gets the credit.

● ● ●

I suspect that we, like the lady in the suite, put a lot of pressure on ourselves to be something significant, and anything that gets in the way of that, or threatens that significance, threatens *us*.

I've noticed, too, that Christians are especially good at wrapping our significance in Christian terms, in ministry terms, to avoid the impression that we're self-centered. But it's still about us. We're not content in what God has done and is doing, and we want the Big Story to include us in a starring role.

> **Christians are especially good at wrapping our significance in Christian terms, in ministry terms, to avoid the impression that we're self-centered.**

Or at least we want to follow someone we think is in a starring role. We like big visionaries, big planners, big, capital-*L* Leaders. (Maybe this explains why, in Christian bookstores, there are frequently ten times as many books on "leadership" than about following.[4] Given that we are called to be disciples and follow, that's a little awkward.) There's just more cachet there. We want to be significant.

The Bible, on the other hand, is shockingly devoid of Awesome, Big Planner-People. Instead, God continually chooses the least likely to be chosen, the broken and the humble. It's clearly His modus operandi.

I've heard this response from people when I talk about this idea: "But how can we possibly get things done without big-time visionaries? Without massive plans to save the world?"

Well, the Bible actually singles out a specific, heroic animal species to illustrate how to get things done. If you want to know how to do it, don't go to the soaring eagle. Don't go to the impressive, roaring lion, either. God may have a different idea:

> Go watch the ants, you lazy person. Watch what they do and be wise. Ants have no commander, no leader or ruler, but they store up food in the summer and gather their supplies at harvest. (Prov. 6:6–8 NCV)

Yes. Watch how the ants operate. They get it.

Sure enough, modern research shows just how remarkable ants are. They all know what to do and when to do it. They know when to rest, when to battle intruders, when to take care of their eggs, all of it. If there are too many ants foraging, just enough ants decide to quit foraging and take on other jobs.

They know how to build massive anthills that are marvels of construction engineering.

And they do it all without a hierarchy. They manage it all without management. They get it done without any one ant knowing the "big picture." No ant is a superstar. No ant is irreplaceable. How they operate is still somewhat mysterious to science, but scientists do know that ants just use the information that's in front of them, and then they respond. That's it. That's all the information an ant has.

The Bible singles out a species wherein every individual member does whatever needs doing, just by responding to what's in front of it. An ant can't worry about the big blueprint. No ant actually has the big picture. *If they each do their thing, the thing right in front of them, the big picture takes care of itself.*

I can't help but think, as much as we humans value our visionaries, that God loves the way the humble ant operates. And as in the case of the young couple who designed a website because they wanted to help some people they loved, it's God who has the Big Picture.

I also can't help but think that if we just responded to things God places in front of us in our lives, and entrusted the visionary role to the Lord Himself, beautiful things could happen. It doesn't mean we don't need leaders; of course we do. But we need humble ones, leaders who don't need a spotlight, don't need approval, and don't need attention. "Ant" leaders who prod us on and serve us in order to help free us to do what God puts in front of us.

I get the impression from reading the stories of the Bible that God really enjoys making marvelous things happen, using the humble. I think it's because then it's obvious who, exactly, made that marvelous thing happen. If anything wonderful happens in my life, and I'm humble, it'll be apparent that it didn't happen because Brant is an amazing visionary. It happened because God will use *anybody* with a willing heart.

And when people look at what happened, they won't walk away feeling disempowered because they'll never be as awesome and talented as I am. Instead, they'll be encouraged to serve God boldly, because, again, He used Brant, so He'll use anybody!

Of course, humility is not about timidity, and it's not about self-denigration. I love C. S. Lewis's description:

To even get near [humility], even for a moment, is like a drink of cold water to a man in a desert.

Do not imagine that if you meet a really humble man he will be what most people call "humble" nowadays: he will not be a sort of greasy, smarmy person, who is always telling you that, of course, he is nobody.

Probably all you will think about him is that he seemed a cheerful, intelligent chap who took a real interest in what *you* said to *him*.

If you do dislike him it will be because you feel a little envious of anyone who seems to enjoy life so easily. He will not be thinking about humility: he will not be thinking about himself at all.[5]

People like that are difficult to offend. When we choose, ahead of time—before conversations, before meetings, before our day begins—to be unoffendable, we're simply choosing humility.

And while, yes, anger happens, as we discussed earlier, it happens so much *less* for people whose egos are not inflamed and who have so little to lose or gain from the approval of others.

Humility means there's so much less at stake, so much less to protect.

You'll become difficult to offend simply because there's so much less of you to defend. When you are headed into a stressful social situation, with difficult, offensive people, and you decide in advance, "I'm not going to let these people

When we choose, ahead of time— before conversations, before meetings, before our day begins—to be unoffendable, we're simply choosing humility.

offend me; I'm forgiving them in advance," you are dying to yourself. You are sacrificing yourself on their behalf. You are making yourself less. You're willingly giving up your own interests and desires, because of your conviction about who Jesus is.

And Jesus tells us there's a reward for this: "Those who want to save their lives will give up true life, and those who give up their lives for me will have true life" (Matt. 16:25 NCV).

At the beginning of this book, we talked about the crazy idea that we are not entitled to anger, and how taking this idea seriously actually opens up new dimensions of rest, grace, and simplicity in our lives. We are, above all, embracing a radical humility.

We're denying ourselves, doing something seemingly self-negating, and then finding that, just as Jesus promised, we haven't lost anything. We've only gained life.

●　●　●

Sokreaksa Himm is an extreme example. He's a Cambodian man whose story is one of the most horrific I've ever heard. He came from a large family, and watched them all die. In 1977, they were beaten to death in front of him, with machetes and hoes. He was fourteen when it happened, and the killers thought they'd killed him too. They left him for dead, buried in a mass grave with thirteen members of his family. His escape is a remarkable story, and his desire for vengeance was every bit as powerful as the grief for his family, he says. He swore himself to it. I'll let you read one of his books (the one I read was *The Tears of My Soul*) and find out about how he became a believer in Jesus. But one of the breathtaking aspects of this, to me, was how quickly he realized he couldn't be a believer in

Jesus and remain angry with his family's killers. He realized it was simply incompatible.

As for me, I grew up surrounded by Jesus-and-Bible talk and church culture, and have been told how anger is vital and even good for us. I was taught how to rationalize my entitlement to it. And yet, a man who's endured the most nightmarish crime imaginable, with limited exposure to Jesus growing up, realized the incompatibility of his burning anger with a Jesus who commands us to forgive.

He realized he couldn't be a believer in Jesus and remain angry with his family's killers. He realized it was simply incompatible.

> For years I cultivated elaborate fantasies in which I tortured and murdered the killers again and again, projecting all my rage and pain I bottled inside myself in my plans for what I would do to the men when I found them. I realized that I would never know true peace until I had dealt with this as well. I had to find a way of forgiving them, before the bitterness inside destroyed me.[6]

Bitterness, anger—he knew he had to get rid of them, even in the face of extreme injustice. If anyone's entitled to "righteous anger," it's Sokreaksa Himm. He'd been raised to believe in it. But with a new nature in Christ, he realized he didn't have a right to such a thing.

> I eventually found two of the men involved in my family's deaths, in the very village and among the very people they terrorized over two decades before. Initially on hearing that

I wanted to meet the men to forgive them, many people thought that my plan was just another attempt to locate the men so that I could take my revenge. To the surprise of the men and most of the villagers, I shook hands with the two men and forgave them.[7]

Self-forgetfulness is not about mystically wishing myself into nonexistence or pretending I'm meaningless. It's just the opposite. Self-forgetfulness is what happens when we're emotionally healthy. It's remembering that God is my defender, His opinion is what matters, and whatever my offenders are doing to me, I've done to others as well. And God has forgiven me. I simply must forgive in return and forfeit my right to anger.

So it's not about "clearing the mind" or embracing nothingness. On the contrary; rather than clearing my mind, I have to remind myself of those larger truths. I have to consider others better than myself, consider how the lilies of the field don't worry about themselves.

Consider.

Remind myself.

Remember that, ultimately, there's something greater happening, a deeper story at work in the world, and at work in me.

24

AND LO, THE KINGDOM OF GOD IS LIKE A TERRIBLE FOOTBALL TEAM

My son is like me. He's not much into athletics. But we signed him up for a flag-football league when he was in sixth grade. My wife told me the league needed someone to coach my son's team, the Rams, and I told her, point-blank, I would not be doing it. I know nothing about coaching football. Nothing. "I will not be coaching the Rams," I said.

The park district called me before the first practice and told me about the Rams, and how they needed a coach, and would I do it? I told them no. "I'm sorry; I just can't do that; it's out of the question. I will not be coaching the Rams."

I dropped Justice off at practice, and all the teams went to different parts of the practice fields. They all had coaches. The

Rams assembled, and everyone's parents had dropped them off, and I towered over all the kids. They asked me if I was their coach. I told them no. "I'm sorry, I will play catch right now, but I will not be coaching the Rams."

The smallest kid, a little scraggly-blonde kid named Jared, threw the ball back and forth with me. He asked me again if I would coach. I told him, again, no. They'd have to find someone else to coach the Rams.

He caught the ball, stopped, and looked at me. He said, "Okay, but for today, can I please call you 'Coach'?"

When I got home, I had to tell my wife why I was carrying a big bag of footballs, pylons, and flags. I was now coaching the Rams.

I was clueless. Over the first eight games, we not only didn't win; we didn't score any points. We were shut out, every game. I loved the kids, but I just didn't know what I was doing. We'd all look over during our practices and see the Yellow Shirt Team Over There, the team that had six football dads, coaching positions, fancy drills, and football-y things I didn't know about. They were amazing, a well-oiled machine. I feared playing them.

We stunk. I think we hit rock bottom when we were penalized for wearing illegal shorts. (Apparently, you can't wear shorts with pockets in flag football.) To avoid forfeiture, I sent my team into the crowd of parents to randomly ask people if they could swap shorts with them. That was a low point.

And we played that team, the Yellow Shirt Team Over There, the one with the dads with visors and whistles and multiple future NCAA recruits, the very last game of the season.

We were 0-11. They were 11-0. Sounds like we had no chance,

right? Sounds like there's no way in the world we could possibly beat these guys, right? They laughed at us before the game.

Something incredible happened. Our best player, a little guy named Christian, returned the opening kickoff for a touchdown. We were ahead 6-0!

So the team that supposedly "didn't have a chance," the one that was mocked, derided, considered the worst-coached team in the league, *now led the game over the mighty Yellow Team!* There were gasps from the crowd. Could the impossible happen? This could be like the 1980 hockey upset, the "Miracle on Ice," all over again. Unbelievable.

I patrolled the sidelines, proudly announcing our intent to go for two!

And then we missed that, and then they scored 77 unanswered points, and we lost 77-6.

So, yeah, it's not really that great of a story.

Except for one thing. As our dejected, winless kids left the field, the kids who went 0-12 and just got humiliated again, something wonderful happened, something you usually don't see in football.

A white stretch limousine pulled up along the field, a limo with flags. Rams flags.

Everyone stopped and stared. The Rams, the playoff-bound Yellow Team, everybody. And a mom said, "Guys, it's time for your end-of-season party!"

The Rams went from dejected losers to royalty. Just like that. They were smiling and laughing and jumping up and down. They all piled into the limo, and off they went for our big pizza-and-swim party.

The Yellow Team, coaches and all, were in awe.

This is how the kingdom of God works. The last are first, the first are last, and in the end, as much as we want to think our performance is all that matters, the victory has exactly nothing to do with us.

We're human, so we're going to occasionally feel threatened. It happens. Anger happens too. So do jealousy and bitterness and resentment. But if you want to be a citizen of this other kingdom, the one in which God promises things will be set right in the end, you may as well remind yourself of it all the time.

The things you think matter so much? They don't matter so much.

The things you think matter so much? They don't matter so much. If you put your trust in God, you're already a "success" because Jesus succeeded. You needn't be insecure in who you are—not because you're so great, but because your security isn't found in who you are.

In the end, you're free to fail all you want, kids, because here's a sweet thought:

The limo is coming for you anyway.

● ● ●

So let's review: Choosing to be unoffendable means choosing to be humble. Not only that, the practice *teaches* humility. Once you've decided you can't control other people; once you've reconciled yourself to the fact that the world, and its people, are broken; once you've realized your own moral failure before God; once you've abandoned the idea that your significance comes from anything other than God, you're growing in humility, and that's exactly where God wants us all.

It's contrary to seemingly everything in our culture, but the more we divest ourselves of ourselves, the better our lives get. Jesus told us as much. He said if we'd give up our lives, for His sake, we'd find real life.

When we surrender our perceived "rights," when we let go of our attempts to manipulate, we find—surprise!—joy.

I've seen it happen in my own life, in little bits. I'm still learning. But I'm so glad someone told me to choose to be unoffendable, because something clicked in my understanding of what it means to follow Jesus. It turns out that life is not only more joy-filled for me but more attractive to others.

I have to die to myself. What I'm finding is it doesn't happen all at once, and it's simultaneously simple to understand and arduous to actually do. But little by little, I think I'm seeing what God is up to.

He wants to be in control. And you know what? I want Him to be. This hasn't always been the case. I think I can trust Him. I don't need to control things anymore. There's so much less at stake when I let go, so much less of me to defend, so much less of "my way" to get in the way and feed my anger.

What a relief. God tells us to die to ourselves, and get rid of anger, for a reason: He loves us.

And I guess I always knew that, that He loves us. But I'm now less prone to anger, and more prone to forgive, because I'm finally really believing, a bit more, day by day, that He actually loves *me*.

Why am I so stressed? Why do I need to pretend I can

control people? Why do I need to make myself "significant"? Why do I think I need to assess other people spiritually? Why am I always trying to assess myself spiritually? Why do I need to defend myself?

God is my Defender. He's in control. And no, I don't know where I'm going, but I know He loves me.

●　●　●

When we lived in Houston, our kids were little, and going anywhere was a logistical nightmare. I remember, one Saturday, finally getting our kids ready to go and buckled into their seats.

We had to stop by the grocery store, so I waited in the car with the kids while Carolyn jumped out, bought her stuff, and jumped back in. We drove around some more, through another neighborhood, to drop something off at some friends'. And then we had a couple more errands to run.

We finally pulled onto I-59 south and drove for about twenty minutes in what I thought was a 65 zone. But it wasn't; it was 55. I got pulled over by a Harris County officer, and we all sat in the car until he came back with a much-deserved ticket.

Eventually we pulled off the shoulder and kept going until we turned onto another interstate. That's when my daughter took her thumb out of her mouth and said something.

"Um . . . Daddy, where are we going?"

Oh. Yeah. I should tell her.

"We're going to the big rodeo. We're going to see horses!"

"Oh! Okay."

That was it. But it dawned on me: How odd had this whole

trip been, from her perspective? From the very outset, she'd just been sitting, buckled in, while we went here and there and everywhere. She'd just watched her mom run in and out, and a strange man approach the car with a funny hat and flashing lights, and we turned this way, and turned that way, and sped up and slowed down and sped up again.

And she had no idea where we were going. None. But she was cool with it.

If that were me, I'd want to know right off the bat. Where are we going? What are we doing? What's up next? Why are we doing this?

But she wasn't the least bit offended with my lack of communication. She's a child, and children are, by nature, humble. They don't have to know everything.

She knew almost nothing—not the distance, not the final destination, not the duration of our stay, not even the reason for leaving her home.

What she did know, though, mattered infinitely. It's the distinctive line between a life of mistrust, stress, exhaustion, anger, bitterness, and ceaseless striving, and a life of contentment and rest. And not just for her but for all of us who know that, ultimately, we're not in control:

She knew who was driving.

She knew, and still knows, that the one who is driving . . . loves her.

And that makes all the difference.

ACKNOWLEDGMENTS

I'm thankful to my wife, Carolyn. She deserves her own paragraph. No one else belongs in her paragraph. This is Carolyn's paragraph.

My son, Justice, in addition to being a blessing in general, helped me getting this book together. My daughter, Julia, made me many coffees at Origin Coffeehouse, where I now sit. Thank you, sweetie. And thank you, mom, dad, step-dad, my dear brother, Darin, and the good people at Thomas Nelson Publishers.

If you ever write a book and think, for even a split-second, that you don't need an editor . . . you're wrong. They see things. Bad things. But then they make them better. (And yes, I know "bad things" is a sentence fragment. But please let that stay.)

Truly, Meaghan Porter and Renee Chavez are brilliant and perceptive. Who knew "Dumpster" had to be capitalized? They did. They know things.

And thank you to our radio show listeners and my Twitter and Facebook friends. Please notice I didn't put "friends" in quotes.

I thank God that I've gotten to be a part of your life, even if just a small one.

NOTES

Epigraph

1. Dallas Willard, "Divine Conspiracy 11: Living Without Anger,"
1:20:59, lecture recorded during the Harvey Fellows 2007 Summer
Institute, posted by "Daniel dliver," June 22, 2011, www.youtube.com
/watch?v=NBBB9G6WW3w.

Chapter 1: Being Unoffendable: The Ridiculous Idea

1. Blaine Smith, "Is Anger a Sin?" Nehemiah Notes, November 15, 2012,
http://www.nehemiahministries.com/isangerasin.htm.
2. Hitendra Wadhwa, "The Wrath of a Great Leader," *Inc.*, January 21,
2013, http://www.inc.com/hitendra-wadhwa/great-leadership-how
-martin-luther-king-jr-wrestled-with-anger.html.

Chapter 2: Everyone's an Idiot but Me

1. Frank Viola, "Living Without Offense," *Beyond Evangelical* (blog),
October 12, 2009, http://frankviola.org/2009/10/12/living-without
-offense-rick-warren-is-supporting-our-twitter-conference-tomorrow/.
2. Dan M. Kahan et al., "Motivated Numeracy and Enlightened

Self-Government," Social Science Research Network, September 8, 2013, https://papers.ssrn.com/sol3/papers.cfm?abstract_id=2319992##.

Chapter 3: Six Billion Rings

1. C. S. Lewis, *Mere Christianity,* rev. and amp. ed. (New York: HarperSanFrancisco, 2009), 93.

Chapter 5: Bert and Ernie and Satan

1. "Neighbors Remember Serial Killer as Serial Killer," *The Onion,* March 5, 1997, http://www.theonion.com/articles /neighbors-remember-serial-killer-as-serial-killer,4357/.

Chapter 6: Beautiful Exceptions

1. M. Night Shyamalan, *The Village,* directed by M. Night Shyamalan (Burbank, CA: Touchstone Pictures, 2004), film.

Chapter 7: The World's Worst Bedtime Story

1. Sheldon Vanauken, *A Severe Mercy* (New York: HarperCollins, 1980).
2. Annie Dillard, *Teaching a Stone to Talk: Expeditions and Encounters* (New York: Harper & Row, 1982), 32.

Chapter 8: Ain't You Tired?

1. *The Help,* directed by Tate Taylor (Universal City, CA: Dreamworks Pictures, 2011), film.

Chapter 10: Idea: Let's Punch Brant in the Face

1. Ericka Sóuter, "10 Most Annoying Gwyneth Paltrow Quotes of All Time," *The Stir* (blog), June 6, 2012, http://thestir.cafemom.com /entertainment/138584/10_most_annoying_gwyneth_paltrow.

Chapter 11: Atheists, Socialists, and Toast

1. Jon Ward, "This Is What Happens When Hip-Hop Lets the Saints In," *Huffington Post,* February 21, 2014, http://www.huffingtonpost .com/2014/02/20/lecrae-moore-rap-christian_n_4784064.html.

2. Mike Yaconelli, *Messy Spirituality* (Grand Rapids, MI: Zondervan, 2002), 54.

3. Ibid. (adapted), 126–27.

Chapter 12: Anger's Fun—Except for the Boiling, Blazing, and Burning Part

1. All of the biblical descriptions of anger that follow are from the New Living Translation.

Chapter 13: The Big Question: What About Injustice?

1. University of British Columbia, "Slacktivism: 'Liking' on Facebook may mean less giving," ScienceDaily, November 8, 2013, http://www.sciencedaily.com/releases/2013/11/131108091320.htm.

2. Arthur C. Brooks, *Who Really Cares: The Surprising Truth About Compassionate Conservatism* (New York: Basic Books, 2007).

3. Christopher A. Hall, "The Gift of Anger," *Christianity Today*, January 1, 2004, http://www.christianitytoday.com/ct/2004/january/28.71.html.

4. Gregory L. Jantz with Ann McMurray, "When Is It OK to Be Angry?" (book excerpt), CBN, http://www.cbn.com/entertainment/books/jantz-guide-to-managing-anger.aspx.

5. Dallas Willard, "Divine Conspiracy 11: Living Without Anger," 1:20:59, lecture recorded during the Harvey Fellows 2007 Summer Institute, posted by "Daniel dliver," June 22, 2011, www.youtube.com/watch?v=NBBB9G6WW3w.

6. Clayborne Carson, ed., *The Autobiography of Martin Luther King, Jr.* (New York: Warner, 1998), 70.

7. Ibid., 80.

8. Dietrich Bonhoeffer, *The Cost of Discipleship*, 1st Touchstone ed. (New York: Touchstone, 1995), 127.

Chapter 14: This Is the Chapter About How We're Just Barely Smart Enough to Be Stupid

1. Robert Sapolsky, *Why Zebras Don't Get Ulcers* (New York: Henry Holt, 2004).

2. Sapolsky, "The Uniqueness of Humans" (Stanford University, September 2009), TED video, 37:26, http://www.ted.com/talks /robert_sapolsky_the_uniqueness_of_humans.

3. Timothy Keller, *King's Cross: The Story of the World in the Life of Jesus* (London: Hodder & Stoughton, 2011), 145.

4. C. S. Lewis, *The Great Divorce* (New York: HarperCollins, 2001), 75.

5. Elise Solé, "Model Cameron Russell: 'Models Are the Most Physically Insecure Women on the Planet,'" Yahoo! Shine, February 1, 2013, https://shine.yahoo.com/fashion-beauty /model-cameron-russell---models-are-the-most-physically -insecure-women-on-the-planet---183444067.html.

Chapter 15: Nothing Left to Lose

1. Judson W. Van DeVenter, "I Surrender All," 1896.

Chapter 16: And Here's the Chapter I Kept Putting Off . . .

1. Brennan Manning, *The Ragamuffin Gospel: Good News for the Bedraggled, Beat-Up, and Burnt Out* (Sister, OR: Multnomah Books, 1990), 29.

2. Charles Wesley, "And Can It Be That I Should Gain," 1739.

Chapter 17: We're All Waiting for Something . . . That Already Happened

1. Khaled Hosseini, *And the Mountains Echoed* (New York: Riverhead, 2013), Kindle version, loc 1435–37.

2. Laurence Bergreen, *Over the Edge of the World: Magellan's Terrifying Circumnavigation of the Globe* (New York: HarperCollins, 2004), 325.

Chapter 18: On Winning—and by "Winning," I Mean, of Course, Losing

1. D. A. Carson, *Love in Hard Places* (Wheaton, IL: Crossway, 2002), 61.

Chapter 21: I Can Worship a God Like That

1. Tony Campolo, *The Kingdom of God Is a Party: God's Radical Plan for His Family* (Nashville: Thomas Nelson, 1990), 5–6.

2. Ibid., 8.

3. Henri Nouwen, *Gracias: A Latin American Journal*, repr. (New York: Harper & Row, 1983; Maryknoll, NY: Orbis, 1993), 147–48. Citations refer to the Orbis edition.

Chapter 22: Here's the Part Where I Talk About Some Danish People

1. Karen Blixen and Gabriel Axel, *Babette's Feast*, directed by Gabriel Axel (Panorama Film A/S, 1987), film.

2. Philip Yancey, *What's So Amazing About Grace?* (Grand Rapids, MI: Zondervan, 1997).

3. Blixen and Axel, *Babette's Feast*.

Chapter 23: Forget Danish People—Let's Talk About Your Elbow

1. Timothy Keller, "Peace—Overcoming Anxiety" (sermon), Timothy Keller Podcast, accessed March 2, 2014, https://itunes.apple.com/us /podcast/peace-overcoming-anxiety/id352660924?i=146253976&mt=2.

2. Thomas Gilovich, Kenneth Savitsky, and Victoria Husted Medvec, "The Spotlight Effect in Social Judgment: An Egocentric Bias in Estimates of the Salience of One's Own Actions and Appearance," *Journal of Personality and Social Psychology* 78, no. 2 (2000): 211–22.

3. Brant Hansen, "Submitted for Your Approval," *Letters from Kamp Krusty* (blog), accessed June 26, 2014, http:// branthansen.typepad.com/letters_from_kamp_krusty /things_im_probably_saying_to_make_the_uncle_jessie_jokes_stop/.

4. Lance Ford, *Unleader* (Kansas City: Beacon Hill, 2013), 26.

5. C. S. Lewis, *Mere Christianity* (New York: Touchstone, 1996), 121.

6. Sokreaksa S. Himm, *The Tears of My Soul* (London: Monarch, 2003), 114.

7. "Sokreaksa Himm (Cambodia)," The Forgiveness Project, October 22, 2012, http://theforgivenessproject.com/stories /sokreaksa-himm-cambodia.

ABOUT THE AUTHOR

Brant Hansen is a radio host who has won multiple National Personality of the Year awards. He also works with CURE International, a worldwide network of hospitals that brings life-changing medical care and the good news of God's love to children with treatable conditions. Brant has been a game inventor and a youth pastor, and is still a very poor (his words) accordion player, although he ardently defends his right to play it.

Brant currently lives in Northern California with his wife, Carolyn; his son, Justice; and his daughter, Julia.

He can be found at branthansen.com and @branthansen on Twitter.